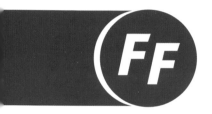

FAST FACTS

FF

*Indispensable
Guides to
Clinical
Practice*

D1482594

Ankylosing spondylitis

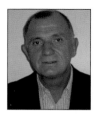

Maxime Dougados MD

Professor of Rheumatology

Hôpital Cochin

René Descartes University

Paris, France

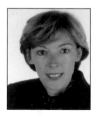

Désirée van der Heijde MD PhD

Professor of Rheumatology

University Hospital Maastricht

Maastricht, The Netherlands

This book is as balanced and as practical as we can make it. Ideas for improvements are always welcome: feedback@fastfacts.com

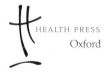

HEALTH PRESS
Oxford

Fast Facts – Ankylosing spondylitis
First published April 2004

Text © 2004 Maxime Dougados, Désirée van der Heijde

© 2004 in this edition Health Press Limited
Fast Facts is a trademark of Health Press Limited,
Elizabeth House, Queen Street, Abingdon,
Oxford OX14 3JR, UK
Tel: +44 (0)1235 523233
Fax: +44 (0)1235 523238

Book orders can be placed via the website or by telephone:
www.fastfacts.com; UK orders 01752 202301; US orders 800 538 1287.

All rights reserved. No part of this publication may be reproduced, stored in a
retrieval system, or transmitted in any form or by any means, electronic, mechanical,
photocopying, recording or otherwise, without the express permission of the
publisher.

The rights of Maxime Dougados and Désirée van der Heijde to be identified as the
authors of this work have been asserted in accordance with the Copyright, Designs
& Patents Act 1988 Sections 77 and 78.

The publisher and the authors have made every effort to ensure the accuracy of this
book, but cannot accept responsibility for any errors or omissions.

Registered names, trademarks, etc. used in this book, even when not marked as such,
are not to be considered unprotected by law.

A CIP catalogue record for this title is available from the British Library.

ISBN 1-903734-44-4

Dougados, M (Maxime)
Fast Facts – Ankylosing spondylitis/
Maxime Dougados, Désirée van der Heijde

Typesetting and page layout by Zed, Oxford, UK.
Printed by Fine Print (Services) Ltd, Oxford, UK.

Printed with vegetable inks on fully biodegradable and
recyclable paper manufactured from sustainable forests.

444   001
Low emissions
during production

Low
chlorine

Sustainable
forests

Glossary

Acute anterior uveitis: inflammation of the ciliary body and iris. This is the most frequent extra-articular manifestation of ankylosing spondylitis, with 25–40% of patients experiencing one or more episodes. The patient typically presents with unilateral eye pain and redness, photophobia and increased lacrimation.

Ankylosis: stiffening or fixation of a joint as a consequence of ossification of the ligaments and also, at the thoracic level, the vertebrocostal and sternocostal joints. The principal concern in patients with spondylitis is progression towards ankylosis. Physical examination reveals impaired spinal mobility, with restricted flexion and extension of the lumbar spine or limited chest expansion.

Anterior chest wall pain: pain that occurs in about 15% of patients and is usually the result of sternoclavicular, manubriosternal or sternocostal arthritis.

Appendicular joints: hip and shoulder. Can be the site of arthritis in ankylosing spondylitis. Hip arthritis often has severe functional consequences.

Axial involvement: involvement of the spine – cervical, thoracic and lumbar – in the disease process. Arthritis of the hip and shoulder and anterior chest wall pain are usually considered as part of axial involvement.

Dactylitis: inflammation of the fingers or toes; in ankylosing spondylitis, the finger or toe takes on a typical 'sausage-like' appearance.

Entheses: the sites of bony insertion of ligaments and tendons.

Enthesitis: painful inflammation of entheses, the sites of bony insertion of ligaments and tendons; this is a classic and frequent feature of ankylosing spondylitis. The most typical enthesitis is inflammatory heel pain (posterior or inferior), which is related to enthesitis of the Achilles tendon or the plantar fascia insertion.

ESSG: European Spondylarthropathy Study Group; this group of experts set up the ESSG criteria for the classification of spondylarthropathies.

Sacroiliitis: inflammation of the sacroiliac joint; the resulting sacroiliac pain is typical of spondylarthropathies.

Peripheral involvement: arthritis of the peripheral joints is mostly oligoarticular, asymmetrical, transient and migratory, with involvement of both small and large joints, predominantly of the lower limbs. It usually appears non-erosive on X-rays.

Prevalence: the percentage of people with the disease in a given population; the reported prevalence of ankylosing spondylitis among adults is 0.1–1.4% in Caucasian populations and 0.04–6% in non-Caucasian populations.

TNFα blockers: tumor necrosis factor alpha blockers; infliximab and etanercept are the two major agents in this class with demonstrated efficacy in treating ankylosing spondylitis.

Twins concordance rate: ratio of the number of pairs with both twins affected over the total number of pairs studied.

Introduction

Désirée van der Heijde and Maxime Dougados

Ankylosing spondylitis is the most typical of the spondylarthropathies, a family of inflammatory diseases that involve the spine and which have an overall prevalence of about 1%. Ankylosing spondylitis onsets in early adulthood and has a major influence on the patient's well-being and physical functioning; it also has an impact on society in general.

The recent availability of effective treatment has increased interest in all aspects of the disease tremendously. This handbook is written for health professionals who want to increase and update their knowledge of this disorder. We provide an overview of the clinical features and diagnosis of ankylosing spondylitis, and discuss what is known about the genetic basis of the disease. The burden of illness on society is also outlined.

We then summarize the management of ankylosing spondylitis, including physical therapy, non-steroidal anti-inflammatory agents, disease-modifying drugs and recently developed biological agents. The closing chapter presents our thoughts on future directions of investigations and management of the disease.

We hope that you find the information practical and easily accessible, and that it helps you to manage your patients with ankylosing spondylitis.

1 The spectrum of spondylarthropathies

Laure Gossec and Maxime Dougados

Ankylosing spondylitis is one of a family of interrelated disorders sharing clinical and genetic characteristics distinct from those of rheumatoid arthritis. The concept of such a family of disorders, called spondylarthropathies, was first introduced by Moll et al. in 1974. The original group of spondylarthropathies included:

- ankylosing spondylitis (the most typical form of spondylarthropathy)
- Reiter's syndrome or reactive arthritis
- arthritis associated with psoriasis, Crohn's disease and ulcerative colitis
- a form of juvenile chronic arthritis.

In 1991, the European Spondylarthropathy Study Group (ESSG) added some less clearly defined disorders, categorized as undifferentiated spondylarthropathies.

Definitive classification of these various forms, especially in the early stages of the disease, is not always possible because of their overlapping clinical features. However, lack of differentiation does not usually affect treatment decisions.

It was noted that several of the spondylarthropathies could occur either sequentially in the same patient or within a family. This suggested a genetic component to these diseases, which was confirmed by a high prevalence of human leukocyte antigen B27 (HLA-B27) not only in patients with ankylosing spondylitis but also in those with other spondylarthropathies.

The primary pathological sites include:

- entheses, which are the sites of bony insertion of ligaments and tendons
- sacroiliac joints and the axial skeleton
- limb joints
- some non-articular structures, such as the gut, skin, eye and aortic valve.

Symptoms may be widespread, but the sites most often affected are the axial skeleton and the lower extremities.

Thus, the spondylarthropathies constitute a cluster of interrelated and overlapping chronic inflammatory rheumatic diseases, which have an uncertain etiology but involve a genetic component. The concept of spondylarthropathy is useful in:

- estimating the prevalence of a group of related disorders that can sometimes be difficult to differentiate from each other
- allowing a diagnosis of spondylarthropathy to be made, which assists in treatment decisions
- allowing a label to be put to the undifferentiated forms, which benefits the patient's psychological status as well as avoiding excessive costly investigations
- monitoring patients, using tools and indexes validated for spondylarthropathies
- determining prognosis
- researching these disorders.

Diagnosis

Spondylarthropathies may sometimes be relatively mild and many patients do not seek medical advice. This, combined with the insidious nature of spondylarthropathies, often precludes an early diagnosis. Many patients are referred several times for the same symptoms without a correct diagnosis being reached. This not only results in prolonged diagnostic delay, but also in many unnecessary and invasive investigations.

Table 1.1 shows the characteristic features of spondylarthropathies. Diagnosis is based on the clinical presentation, association with HLA-B27 and typical radiographic lesions. There are two sets of classification criteria for spondylarthropathies: Amor's criteria and the ESSG criteria (Tables 1.2 and 1.3). The ESSG criteria are more commonly used because they encompass a wider spectrum of disease. Both sets of criteria have been validated by various groups, and their sensitivity and specificity have usually been found to exceed 85%.

However, there is some concern about how useful these diagnostic criteria are in daily clinical practice. They have been derived from trials conducted in patients seen at a late stage of the disease, so may be less useful in those with milder disease and/or those seen at an early stage.

TABLE 1.1

Features of spondylarthropathies

- Radiographic sacroiliitis with or without accompanying spondylitis
- Variable inflammatory peripheral arthritis, enthesitis and dactylitis
- Association with chronic inflammatory bowel disease
- Association with psoriasis and other mucocutaneous lesions
- Tendency towards anterior ocular inflammation
- Increased familial incidence
- Occasional aortitis and heart block
- No association with rheumatoid factor
- Strong association with HLA-B27

Ongoing studies are therefore evaluating the diagnostic use of these classification criteria in patients suffering from a single symptom (e.g. heel pain) at an early stage of the disease. Furthermore, some clinical trials use healthy subjects as the control group and some use other patients referred to a rheumatology clinic. Criteria developed from comparisons with health controls may be less useful in daily practice, where it is likely that the physician will be trying to differentiate between a spondylarthropathy and other rheumatological diagnoses.

Clinical features of spondylarthropathies

Spondylarthropathies can present with a wide spectrum of clinical features. Certain features occur more commonly in some types of spondylarthropathies than others. Typical patterns are shown in Table 1.4. However, it is possible for any of the principal clinical features to be present in any of the distinct diseases.

Psoriatic arthritis. Moll and Wright defined psoriatic arthritis as an 'inflammatory arthritis associated with psoriasis, which is usually negative for rheumatoid factor'. However, there are no internationally agreed criteria for the diagnosis of psoriatic arthritis.

Psoriasis is a common skin disease among Caucasians (1–3% prevalence), but uncommon in some other ethnic groups, such as

TABLE 1.2

Amor's classification criteria for spondylarthropathy

		Score
A	**Clinical symptoms or past history of:**	
	1. Lumbar or dorsal pain at night or morning stiffness of lumbar or dorsal spine	1
	2. Asymmetrical oligoarthritis	2
	3. Buttock pain	1
	If alternating buttock pain	2
	4. Sausage-like toe or digit	2
	5. Heel pain or other well-defined enthesopathy	2
	6. Iritis	1
	7. Non-gonococcal urethritis or cervicitis ≤ 1 month before the onset of arthritis	1
	8. Acute diarrhea ≤ 1 month before the onset of arthritis	1
	9. Psoriasis, balanitis or inflammatory bowel disease (ulcerative colitis or Crohn's disease)	2
B.	**Radiological findings**	
	10. Sacroiliitis (bilateral grade 2 or unilateral grade 3)	3
C.	**Genetic background**	
	11. Presence of HLA-B27 and/or family history of ankylosing spondylitis, reactive arthritis, uveitis, psoriasis or inflammatory bowel disease	2
D.	**Response to treatment**	
	12. Clear-cut improvement within 48 hours of non-steroidal anti-inflammatory drug intake or rapid relapse of pain after their discontinuation	2

Total score: a patient is considered to have a spondylarthropathy if the total score is ≥ 6

TABLE 1.3

The European Spondylarthropathy Study Group (ESSG) criteria for spondylarthropathy

- Inflammatory spinal pain

or

- Synovitis (asymmetric, predominantly in lower extremities)

and

- One or more of the following:
  - Family history: first- or second-degree relative with ankylosing spondylitis, psoriasis, acute iritis, reactive arthritis or inflammatory bowel disease
  - Past or present psoriasis, diagnosed by a physician
  - Past or present ulcerative colitis or Crohn's disease, diagnosed by a physician and confirmed by radiography or endoscopy
  - Past or present pain alternating between the two buttocks
  - Past or present spontaneous pain or tenderness on examination of the site of insertion of the Achilles tendon or plantar fascia (enthesitis)*
  - Episode of diarrhea occurring ≤ 1 month before onset of arthritis
  - Non-gonococcal urethritis or cervicitis occurring ≤ 1 month before onset of arthritis
  - Bilateral grade 2–4 sacroiliitis or unilateral grade 3 or 4 sacroiliitis (where grade 0 is normal, 1 possible, 2 minimal, 3 moderate and 4 completely fused [i.e. ankylosed]).

*There may be inflammation of other entheses, but only Achilles and plantar fascia enthesitis form part of the ESSG criteria

Afro-Caribbeans and Native Americans (0–0.3%). It affects men and women equally. Approximately 10% of patients have associated psoriatic arthritis. Psoriasis usually antedates the appearance of arthritis, but onset is contemporaneous in 20% of patients, and in up to 15% the arthritis may precede the onset or diagnosis of psoriasis. The arthritis usually onsets between the ages of 30 and 50 years, but can also begin in childhood. In the majority of patients, exacerbations

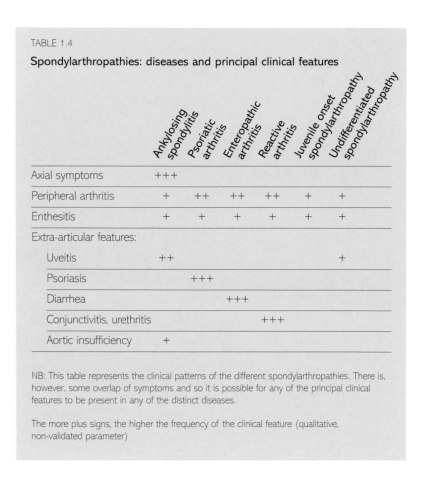

TABLE 1.4

Spondylarthropathies: diseases and principal clinical features

	Ankylosing spondylitis	Psoriatic arthritis	Enteropathic arthritis	Reactive arthritis	Juvenile onset spondylarthropathy	Undifferentiated spondylarthropathy
Axial symptoms	+++					
Peripheral arthritis	+	++	++	++	+	+
Enthesitis	+	+	+	+	+	+
Extra-articular features:						
Uveitis	++					+
Psoriasis		+++				
Diarrhea			+++			
Conjunctivitis, urethritis				+++		
Aortic insufficiency	+					

NB: This table represents the clinical patterns of the different spondylarthropathies. There is, however, some overlap of symptoms and so it is possible for any of the principal clinical features to be present in any of the distinct diseases.

The more plus signs, the higher the frequency of the clinical feature (qualitative, non-validated parameter)

and remissions of skin and joint involvement occur with little or no apparent relationship.

There is a polyarticular or oligoarticular pattern of joint involvement in 90% of patients. Approximately 5% present with predominant spondylitis. A few patients present with predominant distal interphalangeal disease, a mutilating type of disease known as arthritis mutilans or the rare synovitis–acne–pustulosis–hyperostosis–osteomyelitis (SAPHO) syndrome. The typical pattern of joint involvement is an asymmetrical distribution with distal interphalangeal involvement and dactylitis.

Psoriatic arthritis is a chronic erosive disease and treatments resemble those of rheumatoid arthritis.

TABLE 1.5

Bacteria that trigger reactive arthritis

- *Chlamydia trachomatis*
- *Shigella flexneri*
- *Salmonella* spp
- *Yersinia enterolytica*
- *Yersinia pseudotuberculosis*
- *Campylobacter fetus jejuni*
- *Clostridium difficile*
- Intravesical injection of bacille Calmette-Guérin to treat bladder cancer
- *Chlamydia pneumoniae*: unconfirmed

Enteropathic arthritis describes the occurrence of inflammatory arthritis in patients with ulcerative colitis or Crohn's disease. The frequency of arthritis in inflammatory bowel disease ranges from 17% to 20%, with a higher prevalence in patients with Crohn's disease.

The most common manifestation of enteropathic arthritis is inflammation of the peripheral (limb) joints. Axial involvement and enthesitis may also be encountered. The peripheral arthritis is usually transient, migratory and non-deforming. The inflammatory episodes are generally self-limiting, often subsiding within 6 weeks, but recurrences are common. In some cases, the arthritis may become chronic and destructive. Intestinal symptoms usually antedate or coincide with joint manifestations, but arthritis may precede the intestinal symptoms by years.

Reactive arthritis describes an episode of aseptic peripheral arthritis that occurs within 1 month of a primary infection elsewhere in the body, usually a genitourinary infection with *Chlamydia trachomatis* or enteritis due to Gram-negative enterobacteria such as *Shigella*, *Salmonella*, *Yersinia* or *Campylobacter* species (Table 1.5).

It can also follow local injection of bacille Calmette-Guérin (BCG) into the site of bladder cancer, but not BCG inoculation as used in some countries to decrease the risk of tuberculosis. Genitourinary tract infection with *Chlamydia trachomatis* is the most commonly recognized initiator of reactive arthritis in developed countries, whereas infections with enterobacteria are reported to be the most common triggers in developing parts of the world. In about 25% of cases, however, the triggering organism is unknown. Reactive arthritis is classified as a spondylarthropathy because it is linked to HLA-B27 and shares clinical features with other spondylarthropathies.

Reactive arthritis is typically an acute, asymmetric oligoarthritis and is frequently associated with one or more characteristic extra-articular features such as ocular inflammation (conjunctivitis or acute iritis), enthesitis, mucocutaneous lesions, urethritis and, on rare occasions, carditis. Conjunctivitis occurs in one-third of patients with reactive arthritis, usually at the same time as flares of arthritis, and acute anterior uveitis may occur at some time in about 5% of patients. The triad of arthritis, conjunctivitis and urethritis is called Reiter's syndrome; most patients with reactive arthritis do not present with this triad.

Treatment of reactive arthritis differs from that of other spondylarthropathies because it involves prolonged antibiotic therapy (although the efficacy of antibiotics remains unproven).

The average duration of the arthritis is 4–5 months, but two-thirds of patients have mild musculoskeletal symptoms that persist for more than 1 year. Recurrent attacks are more common in patients with *Chlamydia*-induced reactive arthritis. Approximately 15–30% of patients develop chronic or recurrent peripheral arthritis, sacroiliitis or spondylitis. Most patients with reactive arthritis have a positive family history for spondylarthropathy or are positive for HLA-B27.

Juvenile-onset spondylarthropathies usually first manifest as peripheral arthritis or enthesitis in children aged 8–12 years, but onset at younger or older ages also occurs. There is a striking predominance of males, particularly in the prepubertal stage. Juvenile-onset spondylarthropathies resemble their adult counterparts, with diverse associations of peripheral arthritis, enthesitis and axial involvement. The disease pattern often changes throughout childhood, adolescence and adulthood (e.g. from monarthritis to a more complex form of disease leading to axial, peripheral and extra-articular manifestations). Oligoarthritis affecting the knee, ankle and/or mid-foot is the typical initial presentation.

There are undifferentiated and differentiated forms of juvenile-onset spondylarthropathies, which can be classified according to the International Associations for Rheumatology criteria in the enthesitis-related-arthritis (ERA) subgroup. The adult ESSG criteria, which have been validated in children, may also be used.

Prognosis is less favorable in juvenile-onset spondylarthropathies than in adult spondylarthropathies. There is the potential for structural damage at some sites (particularly the feet, hips and, sometimes, the spine), leading to functional impairment at long-term follow-up. Nearly 60% of patients have moderate-to-severe limitations 10 years after disease onset. The probability of remission is only 17% after a disease duration of 5 years.

Undifferentiated spondylarthropathies are frequently under-diagnosed and include isolated clinical syndromes, such as HLA-B27-associated seronegative oligoarthritis or polyarthritis, mostly of the lower limbs. This arthritis has no recognizable preceding bacterial infectious trigger, nor associated inflammatory bowel disease or psoriasis. Patients with undifferentiated spondylarthropathy may have dactylitis, with a

---

Key points – the spectrum of spondylarthropathies

- Spondylarthropathies are a heterogeneous family of disorders characterized by the association of:
  - axial inflammatory pain and sometimes ankylosis
  - variable inflammatory peripheral arthritis, predominantly asymmetrical and affecting the lower limbs
  - enthesitis (e.g. heel pain).
- They may be associated with extra-articular features such as chronic inflammatory bowel disease, psoriasis, urethritis and a tendency to anterior ocular inflammation.

sausage-like appearance to the affected finger or toe. They may also experience enthesitis, especially at the heel. Some patients may present with an episode of acute anterior uveitis (acute iritis) or have a syndrome of aortic incompetence plus heart block. The cardiac syndrome or the acute iritis may occur in patients who never develop signs of arthritis, and may sometimes accompany or precede the onset of spondylarthropathy.

Key references

Amor B, Dougados M, Mijiyawa M. Critères de classification des spondylarthropathies. *Rev Rhum Mal Ostéoart* 1990;57:85–9.

Amor B, Santos RS, Nahal R et al. Predictive factors of the long-term outcome of spondyloarthropathies. *J Rheumatol* 1994;21:1883–7.

Calin A. The material history and prognosis of ankylosing spondylitis. *J Rheumatol* 1985;15:1054–5.

Dougados M, Hochberg MC. Why is the concept of spondyloarthropathies important? *Best Pract Res Clin Rheumatol* 2002;16:495–505.

Dougados M, van der Linden S, Juhlin R et al. The European Spondylarthropathy Study Group preliminary criteria for the classification of spondyloarthropathy. *Arthritis Rheum* 1991;34:1218–30.

Keat A. Reiter's syndrome and reactive arthritis in perspective. *N Engl J Med* 1983;309:1606–15.

Khan MA, van der Linden SM. A wider spectrum of spondyloarthropathies. *Semin Arthritis Rheum* 1990;20:107–13.

Leirisalo-Repo M, Turunel U, Steinman S et al. High frequency of silent inflammatory bowel disease in spondyloarthropathy. *Arthritis Rheum* 1994;37:23–31.

Mielants H, Veys EM, Cuvelier C, de Vos M. Course of gut inflammation in spondylarthropathies and therapeutic consequences. *Bailliere's Clin Rheumatol* 1996;10:147–64.

Moll JM, Haslock I, Macrae IF, Wright V. Associations between ankylosing spondylitis, psoriatic arthritis, Reiter's disease, the intestinal arthropathies and Behçet's syndrome. *Medicine* (Baltimore) 1974;53:343–64.

Moll JM, Wright V. Psoriatic arthritis. *Semin Arthritis Rheum* 1973;3:55–78.

Sieper J, Rudwaleit M, Braun J, van der Heijde D. Diagnosing reactive arthritis: role of clinical setting in the value of serologic and microbiologic assays. *Arthritis Rheum* 2002;46:319–27.

van der Linden SJ, van der Heijde D. Ankylosing spondylitis. *Rheum Dis Clin North Am* 1998;24:663–915.

Corinne Miceli-Richard and Maxime Dougados

Genetic risk factors for ankylosing spondylitis were suspected for a long time because of the frequent familial clustering of cases. The first genetic factor to be identified was HLA-B27. Further genetic epidemiological studies have suggested the existence of other predisposing genes. Recent progress on genome sequencing will facilitate their identification.

HLA-B27

The existence of genetic susceptibility factors for ankylosing spondylitis was first suggested between 1950 and 1960. An association between HLA-B27 and ankylosing spondylitis was reported in 1973, both by Schlosstein and by Brewerton. Schlosstein, from the University of California, observed HLA-B27 in 88% of ankylosing spondylitis patients and only 6% of healthy controls. At the same time, Brewerton, from the London Westminster Hospital, found that 95% of patients with ankylosing spondylitis had HLA-B27. Further investigations in the 1990s on B27-transgenic rats confirmed that B27 is directly involved in susceptibility to ankylosing spondylitis.

Although it is clear that HLA-B27 is implicated in the pathophysiology of the disease, its exact role remains unknown. Recent evidence suggests that this tissue antigen may not behave like other class 1 histocompatibility molecules. HLA-B27 heavy chains can form homodimers that do not contain the β_2-microglobulin light chain (a phenomenon termed HLA-B27 misfolding). Such homodimers could mediate or be the target of a pro-inflammatory response. This hypothesis is currently under investigation.

Family studies

A large family with multiple cases of ankylosing spondylitis was reported in 1968 by Bremner et al. The researchers found that among currently unaffected members of the family, the risk of developing ankylosing spondylitis was 20–40 times higher than in the general population (computed as the prevalence of the disease among relatives divided by the prevalence of the disease in the general population, i.e. 4% divided by 0.1–0.2%). In the early 1970s, an increasing number of families affected by ankylosing spondylitis was studied. It was observed that HLA-B27 co-segregated with the disease in these families, favoring direct involvement of the HLA-B27 gene in predisposing individuals to the disease. However, Calin and van der Linden demonstrated that this tissue antigen did not wholly account for susceptibility to the disease within affected families, suggesting that other factors, presumably genetic, were involved. The study published in 1984 by van der Linden reported that the risk of developing ankylosing spondylitis was over 15 times higher in B27-carrier first-degree relatives of patient with ankylosing spondylitis (21%) than in B27-carriers in the general population (1.3%).

Twin studies

The difference in concordance between monozygotic and dizygotic twins confirms the importance of genetic factors in predisposing individuals to ankylosing spondylitis. In addition, twin-pair studies have demonstrated that some genetic factors are not linked to the major histocompatibility complex (MHC).

The concordance rate is calculated as the number of pairs with both twins affected divided by the total number of pairs of twins, expressed as a percentage. Since monozygotic twins inherit identical genetic material, the expected concordance rate would be 100% if the disease determinants were purely genetic (Figure 2.1). This is not the case for ankylosing spondylitis, which appears to be a complex disease in which both environmental and genetic factors are involved. In fact, twin-pair studies have reported a monozygotic concordance rate of about 70%, suggesting that as much as 30% of the susceptibility to the disease might be due to environmental factors.

The concordance rate differs between B27-carrier dizygotic twins (about 25%) and B27-positive monozygotic twins (about 70%), suggesting that the genetic component of susceptibility to ankylosing spondylitis cannot be explained solely by HLA-B27 status.

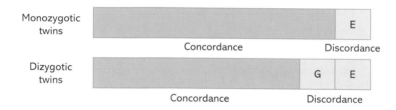

Figure 2.1 Concordance and discordance in monozygotic and dizygotic twins. A pair is concordant if both twins are affected, and is discordant if only one twin is affected. Discordance between monozygotic twins is related to environmental factors (E); discordance between dizygotic twins is of genetic (G) and environmental (E) origin.

Methodology of genetic studies

The genetic analysis of complex multifactorial diseases such as ankylosing spondylitis is challenging. The underlying model of disease inheritance is unknown and it is likely that several genes are involved. Furthermore, the specific genes involved may differ from patient to patient (genetic heterogeneity). In addition, the molecular variant of a gene (i.e. the allele) associated with susceptibility to ankylosing spondylitis may be present in healthy subjects as well as those with the disease, suggesting that exposure to specific environmental factors is required for ankylosing spondylitis to develop (i.e. there is incomplete penetrance). Two main strategies have been used to identify genes that increase susceptibility to ankylosing spondylitis: the candidate gene and the genome scanning approaches.

Candidate gene approach. Certain genes may be regarded as being likely to have a role in the pathophysiology of the disease. In the case of ankylosing spondylitis, genes coding for cytokines and those involved in apoptosis are good candidate genes. Once a candidate gene has been identified, genetic polymorphisms (molecular differences) are analyzed. Some polymorphisms are unlikely to have a functional effect (e.g. those resulting in a conservative amino-acid substitution). Others that affect regulatory regions of the gene or lead

19

to a truncation of the related protein (as has been demonstrated for CARD15, a gene associated with Crohn's disease) are more likely to have a functional influence.

The candidate gene approach is often based on case-control studies that compare the frequency of alleles of a gene in patients and in healthy controls (Figure 2.2). A statistically significant difference in frequency indicates that the allele is associated with the disease. It is important, however, that the control group is carefully defined in order to avoid frequency differences that are not related to the disease. For example, patients and controls should be ethnically matched. In order to overcome this potential bias, specific statistical tests have been developed, such as the transmission disequilibrium test proposed by Spielman. This test analyzes intrafamilial transmission of alleles, but requires genotyping of the patient's parents (Figure 2.3).

Several genes have been investigated as candidate genes for ankylosing spondylitis (Table 2.1). However, many studies have

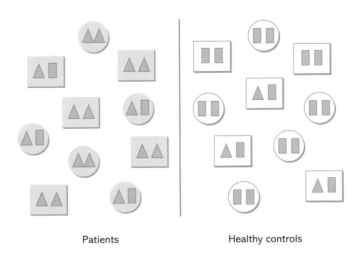

Patients   Healthy controls

Figure 2.2 Association studies: the polymorphic marker tested is bi-allelic. The triangle and oblong alleles are not equally distributed among patients and healthy controls. This suggests that the disease is associated with the triangle allele.

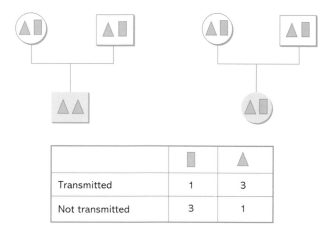

Transmitted	1	3
Not transmitted	3	1

Figure 2.3 Transmission disequilibrium test: the number of alleles transmitted and not transmitted to affected children by their heterozygous parents is calculated for each allele within a family set. An allele involved in the disease pathogenesis is expected to be transmitted in excess to affected offspring.

produced negative results, while others have demonstrated only a weak association. With the exception of HLA-B27, none of the genes studied appear to have a major effect on susceptibility to ankylosing spondylitis.

Genome scanning approach. An alternative strategy is to attempt to localize one or more regions of the genome that may contain genes that increase susceptibility to the disease. Linkage studies are performed in multiplex families (i.e. those with several relatives affected by the disease), using computer software to try to identify genetic resemblance regions in affected family members. Family members are scanned for a panel of 300–400 highly polymorphic markers, called microsatellites, that are evenly distributed throughout the genome. Susceptibility loci are defined by regions that are shared more often by affected individuals than would be expected according to Mendel's law. More refined analysis of these broad genomic regions is then undertaken by a process known as fine mapping, in which a denser set of markers is used.

21

TABLE 2.1

Genes investigated by case-control or intrafamilial association studies in spondylarthropathies

- Androgen receptor
- ANKH (*Homo sapiens* homolog of murine progressive ankylosis)
- CARD15/NOD2 (apoptosis regulator)
- CYP2D6 (debrisoquine hydroxylase)
- HLA-B27 (human leukocyte antigen B27)
- HLA-B60 (human leukocyte antigen B60)
- HLA-DRB1 (human leukocyte antigen DRB1)
- HSP70 (heat shock protein, 70 kD)
- IL-1RA (interleukin-1RA)
- IL-10 (interleukin-10)
- LMP2 (proteasome subunit)
- LMP7 (proteasome subunit)
- MICA (major histocompatibility complex class I related-polypeptide sequence A)
- TAP (transporter associated with antigen processing)
- T-cell receptor
- TNFα (tumor necrosis factor α)

To date, two genome-wide scanning studies in ankylosing spondylitis have been published, both by the same research group from Oxford, UK. Regions of interest have been identified on chromosomes 1, 2, 6 (the MHC region), 9, 10, 16 and 19. The strongest linkage other than the MHC region has been found on chromosome 16q (q denotes the long arm of a chromosome, and p the short arm). Other genome scanning studies are under way in multiplex families identified in France and North America. It is hoped that the results of these linkage studies will enable susceptibility loci to be identified for ankylosing spondylitis.

Key points – genetic aspects

- Individuals with the HLA-B27 tissue antigen have an increased risk of developing ankylosing spondylitis.
- Genetic epidemiological studies suggest the existence of other predisposing genes, though none of the genes studied so far has a strong association with ankylosing spondylitis.
- Genome scanning studies reveal that the strongest linkage, other than the MHC region, is to be found on chromosome 16q.

Key references

Brown MA, Kennedy LG, MacGregor AJ et al. Susceptibility to ankylosing spondylitis in twins. The role of genes, HLA, and the environment. *Arthritis Rheum* 1997; 40:1823–8.

Brown MA, Laval SH, Brophy S, Calin A. Recurrence risk modelling of the genetic susceptibility to ankylosing spondylitis. *Ann Rheum Dis* 2000;59:883–6.

Laval SH, Timms A, Edwards S et al. Whole-genome screening in ankylosing spondylitis: evidence of non-MHC genetic-susceptibility loci. *Am J Hum Genet* 2001;68:918–26.

van der Linden SM, Valkenburg HA, de Jongh BM, Cats A. The risk of developing ankylosing spondylitis in HLA-B27 positive individuals. A comparison of relatives of spondylitis patients with the general population. *Arthritis Rheum* 1984;27:241–9.

Wordsworth P. Genes in the spondyloarthropathies. *Rheum Dis Clin North Am* 1998;24:845–63.

Annelies Boonen and Désirée van der Heijde

Prevalence and incidence

Ankylosing spondylitis occurs worldwide, but its prevalence shows remarkable geographic variation. This can be attributed partly to differences in the prevalence of HLA-B27 in different populations. Moreover, the strength of the association between this tissue antigen and ankylosing spondylitis depends on the subtype of HLA-B27. Up to 25 subtypes have been identified. Subtypes HLA-B*2705 and HLA-B*2704 are strongly associated with the disease, while subtype HLA-B*2706, which occurs in South-East Asia, seems to lack association with ankylosing spondylitis. In addition to genetic predisposition, environmental factors play a role in the development of the disease.

Overall, the reported prevalence of ankylosing spondylitis among adults is 0.1–1.4% in Caucasian populations and 0.04–6% in non-Caucasian populations (Table 3.1). The prevalence of the whole spectrum of the spondylarthropathies, of which ankylosing spondylitis is the typical example, is estimated to be 1.9% among Caucasians, according to a recent study. A population study conducted in Brittany, France, emphasized that the prevalence of the spondylarthropathies was only slightly lower than the prevalence of rheumatoid arthritis.

Ankylosing spondylitis develops in 1–2% of individuals who have HLA-B27 in most Western European and North American societies, but in 6.7% of people with HLA-B27 in Norway. The disease occurs in 10–30% of HLA-B27-positive first-degree relatives of HLA-B27-positive patients

The observed incidence of 7.3/100 000 person-years in the USA is similar to the more recently reported figure of 6.3/100 000 person-years in Finland.

Comorbid conditions. Peripheral arthritis, inflammatory bowel disease, psoriasis and acute anterior uveitis are well-recognized comorbid

TABLE 3.1

Prevalence of ankylosing spondylitis in different populations

Population	Disease prevalence	HLA-B27 prevalence
Caucasian populations		
The Netherlands	0.1%	8%
USA (Minnesota)	0.13%	
Finland	0.15%	
Hungary	0.4%	14%
Germany (Berlin)	0.86%	9.3%
Norway (Oslo)	1.1–1.4%	16%
Non-Caucasian populations		
Japan (adults)	0.04–0.0065%	< 1%
Taiwan	0.19–0.54%	
China	0.26%	4%
Eskimos	0.4%	> 20%
Haida Indians	6%	50%

conditions in patients with ankylosing spondylitis. However, few studies have directly assessed how often these diseases coexist with ankylosing spondylitis. It is generally accepted that up to 25% of patients with ankylosing spondylitis have peripheral arthritis, 20% have clinical inflammatory bowel disease, 8% have psoriasis and 40% have an acute anterior uveitis at some point during the course of disease.

Socioeconomic consequences

Ankylosing spondylitis can impose significant physical limitations on patients, affecting their ability to work and/or reducing their quality of life. This, together with the advent of effective but expensive therapies with biological agents, has led to increased interest in the socioeconomic consequences of the disease. Moreover, ankylosing spondylitis onsets at an early age, typically in the patient's third decade, which increases the lifetime impact of the disease.

Labor force participation. The rate of withdrawal from work among ankylosing spondylitis patients with a paid job is high in Mexico (3% per year), intermediate in Europe (36% after 20 years in a French study and 31% after 20 years in a Dutch study) and low in the USA (10% after 10 years and also after 20 years; Table 3.2). In the Netherlands, the age- and gender-adjusted rate of withdrawal from the labor force is 3.1 times higher in patients with ankylosing spondylitis than in the general population. For comparison, in patients with rheumatoid arthritis in the Netherlands, withdrawal from work is reported to be 50% after 10 years of disease.

Factors associated with a higher risk of work disability among patients with ankylosing spondylitis include older age at disease onset, manual work, and behavioral coping styles characterized by limiting and pacing activities (Figure 3.1). In addition, absence of vocational counseling or job training, difficulty accessing the workplace, and lack of support from colleagues and management all increase the probability of withdrawal from work. Each year in the USA, 15% of ankylosing spondylitis patients in paid jobs take short-term disease-related sick

TABLE 3.2

Withdrawal rate from labor force due to work disability in patients who had a paid job at onset of ankylosing spondylitis

Population*	Withdrawal rate	Comment
Mexico	3% per year	
France	36% after 20 years	
The Netherlands	30% after 20 years	Relative risk compared with the general population: 3.1 (95% confidence interval: 2.5–3.7)
USA	10% after 20 and 30 years	Highly educated patients; individuals with inflammatory bowel disease excluded from study

*n = 103 for Mexico, n = 182 for France, n = 529 for the Netherlands and n = 234 for the USA

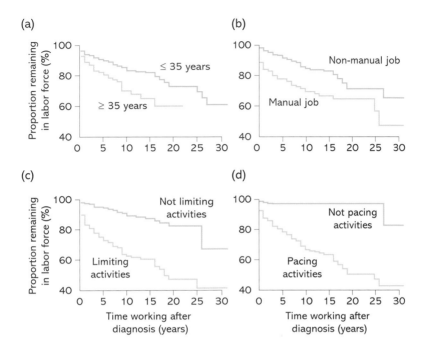

Figure 3.1 There is a higher risk of withdrawal from the labor force because of ankylosing spondylitis in patients who are older at diagnosis, who are in manual as opposed to non-manual jobs, and who adopt limiting (i.e. stopping activity) or pacing styles (i.e. continue activity, but more slowly) of coping with pain. (a) Age at diagnosis; (b) type of work; (c) and (d) behavioral coping styles.

leave; the corresponding figure in Europe is 38%. Ankylosing spondylitis was reported to result in 13 days' absence from work per year per working patient in Europe. The mean number of days of sick leave was associated with disease activity and the presence of extraspinal disease manifestations.

Cost of illness. Classically, the direct healthcare and non-healthcare costs, the productivity costs and the intangible costs are considered in cost-of-illness studies. Table 3.3 compares the cost of ankylosing spondylitis in the USA and Europe.

Direct healthcare and non-healthcare costs. The mean direct costs to society due to ankylosing spondylitis were US$1775 (median US$1113)

TABLE 3.3

Cost of ankylosing spondylitis to society in USA and Europe

	USA (n = 241) US$/patient/year		Europe* (n = 210) €/patient/year**	
	Mean	Median	Mean	Median
Direct healthcare costs	1566	1113	2172 (US$2405)	1002 (US$1109)
Direct non-healthcare costs	209	0	468 (US$518)	104 (US$115)
All direct costs	1775	1113	2640 (US$2923)	1242 (US$1375)
Productivity costs[†]	4945	0	6812 (US$7542)	90 (US$100)
Total costs	6720	1495	9452 (US$10 465)	2894 (US$3204)

*Based on data from the Netherlands, France and Belgium
**US$ are given in brackets for comparative purposes; an exchange rate of
€1 to US$1.1071 applied at the time of the study
[†]Productivity costs calculated using the human capital cost approach, which comprises costs because of sick leave and work disability. The productivity costs account for 74% of total costs in the USA and 72% in Europe

per patient per year in the USA, and €2640 (median €1242) in a European tri-nation study (involving the Netherlands, France and Belgium); at the time of both studies, €1 equated to US$1.1071. In the USA, drugs accounted for the highest proportion of the expenses (41% of total costs), followed by cost of hospitalizations (16%). In Europe, the cost of hospitalizations was the main cost driver (27% of total costs), followed by costs of drugs (13%) and physiotherapy (13%).

In the European study, the mean number of times that a patient with ankylosing spondylitis visited a physiotherapist in a year was 19, compared with only three visits in the US study. Patients in the European study were hospitalized for a mean of 2.3 days per year, compared with 0.06 days in the USA. It is important to note that the US patients were more highly educated, and those with inflammatory bowel disease were excluded from the study. In the European study, the

---

Key points – epidemiology and socioeconomic impact

- The prevalence of ankylosing spondylitis is 0.1–1.4% in Caucasians and 0.04–6% in non-Caucasian populations.
- The rate of withdrawal from the labor force is three times higher in patients with ankylosing spondylitis than in the general population, according to a Dutch study.
- In the USA as well as in Europe, the cost of illness to society incurred by ankylosing spondylitis is substantial; the highest costs were associated with patients who had the greatest degree of physical disability due to the disease.
- The quality of life for patients with ankylosing spondylitis is impaired relative to the general population.
- The benefits of spa treatment for patients with ankylosing spondylitis can be gained at an acceptable average additional cost.

---

highest direct costs were incurred by patients who had longer duration of disease, lower educational level, greater physical limitations and higher disease activity.

Productivity costs. The US and European studies measured annual productivity costs to society as a result of ankylosing spondylitis using the human capital approach, which takes into account both sick leave and work disability. The mean productivity costs were US$4945 per patient (median US$0) in the USA, compared with €6812 (median €90) in the European study. The friction costs (in which the productivity costs to society are calculated on the basis of sick leave only) were assessed in the European study, giving a mean of €465 (median €0) per patient per year. In the USA as well as in Europe, the highest productivity costs to society were incurred by patients who had greater physical limitations.

Intangible costs. Chronic diseases can have an important impact on the quality of life experienced by patients. Such effects are relevant in economic assessments, but are difficult to capture in monetary terms. In a US survey of patients with ankylosing spondylitis, 90% of participants reported stiffness, 83% pain, 63% fatigue and 54% poor sleep. Furthermore, 51% were concerned about their appearance, 51% had worries about the future and 41% expressed concern about the side effects of medication. In the European tri-nation study, quality of life measured by the EQ-5D was lower in patients with ankylosing spondylitis than in subjects with a similar age and gender distribution from the general population.

Full economic evaluations relate the costs of an intervention or a treatment program to its effects. Only one cost-effectiveness study in ankylosing spondylitis has been published. Among 120 Dutch patients, the costs per quality-adjusted life-year (QALY) gained with spa exercise treatment in Austria (group 1) or spa exercise treatment in a local spa resort (group 2) were compared with usual care, which comprised group physical exercises. The cost of spa exercise treatment was €1739 in Austria and €1515 in a local spa resort. In both of the spa treatment groups, cost-savings were noted for medications, visits to physiotherapists and days of sick leave, compared with the usual care group. There was also a positive effect on quality of life in those receiving spa treatment. The incremental cost-utility ratio was €7465 per QALY (95% confidence interval: €3294–14 686) for group 1 and €18 575 per QALY (95% confidence interval: €3678–114 257) for group 2, compared with the usual care group. In Western European countries and North America, these results are considered acceptable cost-effectiveness values.

Key references

Braun J, Bollow M, Remlinger G et al. Prevalence of spondylarthropathies in HLA-B27 positive and negative blood donors. *Arthritis Rheum* 1998;41:58–67.

Boonen A, Chorus A, Miedema H et al. Withdrawal from labour force due to work disability in patients with ankylosing spondylitis. *Ann Rheum Dis* 2001;60:1033–9.

Boonen A, de Vet H, van der Heijde D, van der Linden S. Work status and its determinants among patients with ankylosing spondylitis. A systematic literature review. *J Rheumatol* 2001;28:1056–62.

Boonen A, van der Heijde D, Landewe D et al. Direct costs of ankylosing spondylitis and its determinants. An analysis among three European countries. *Ann Rheum Dis* 2003;62:732–40.

Boonen A, van der Heijde D, Landewe R et al. Work status and productivity costs due to ankylosing spondylitis: comparison of three European countries. *Ann Rheum Dis* 2002;61:429–37.

Chorus AMJ, Boonen A, Miedema HS, van der Linden S. Employment perspectives of patients with ankylosing spondylitis. *Ann Rheum Dis* 2002;61:693–9.

Saraux A, Guedes C, Allain J et al. Prevalence of rheumatoid arthritis and spondylarthropathies in Brittany, France. *J Rheumatol* 1999;26: 2622–7.

Ward M, Kuzis S. Risk factors for work disability in patients with ankylosing spondylitis. *J Rheumatol* 2001;28:315–21.

Ward MM. Functional disability predicts total costs in patients with ankylosing spondylitis. *Arthritis Rheum* 2002;46:223–31.

Laure Gossec and Maxime Dougados

Ankylosing spondylitis may present with a wide spectrum of clinical features characteristic of the spondylarthropathies. In this chapter, we will focus on the most common features of ankylosing spondylitis: axial symptoms, peripheral arthritis, enthesitis and uveitis.

Demographics and diagnostic delay

Ankylosing spondylitis is the most common and most typical form of spondylarthropathy. It is 2–3 times more common in men than women. Although it seldom onsets after 45 years of age, ankylosing spondylitis is often diagnosed at an older age, partly because symptoms may be minimal for years.

A recent survey of 1614 patients with ankylosing spondylitis illustrates the protracted delay between onset and diagnosis. The mean age at disease onset was found to be 25.7 years, and the mean delay in diagnosis was 8.9 years. A significantly greater delay in diagnosis was seen in women than in men (9.8 years versus 8.4 years, $p < 0.01$). This discrepancy in disease detection between the sexes reflects the common problem of underdiagnosis of ankylosing spondylitis among women, probably due to the misconception that only men are affected.

Although no laboratory test is diagnostic for ankylosing spondylitis, the HLA-B27 gene is present in 90–95% of Caucasian patients with this disease in central Europe and North America.

The modified New York criteria for ankylosing spondylitis are commonly used in diagnosis (Table 4.1). They are readily applicable to patients showing clear radiological evidence of the disease, but are of limited use in the absence of defined radiological signs. Many investigators have tried to establish diagnostic criteria for the early stages of ankylosing spondylitis, but none of these has been universally accepted.

TABLE 4.1

Modified New York criteria for diagnosis of ankylosing spondylitis

A definite diagnosis of ankylosing spondylitis can be made if
criterion 4 and any one of the other criteria are fulfilled

1. Low back pain of at least 3 months' duration that is improved by
   exercise and not relieved by rest

2. Limited lumbar spinal motion in sagittal and frontal (anterior and
   posterior) planes

3. Chest expansion decreased relative to normal values for sex
   and age

4. Bilateral sacroiliitis grade 2–4 or unilateral sacroiliitis grade 3 or 4

Axial features

Inflammatory spine pain. Symptoms of ankylosing spondylitis
usually first appear in late adolescence or early adulthood. The
key symptom is inflammatory back pain, often associated with
sacroiliac involvement.

Classically, pain starts in the lumbar region or at the lumbodorsal
junction. It is typically a dull pain of insidious onset, becoming
persistent after a few months. It is inflammatory in nature – the pain
worsens with inactivity, morning stiffness is often prolonged and
nocturnal pain may awaken the patient.

At a later stage, spondylitis may involve the dorsal or cervical spine;
neck pain and stiffness are characteristic of advanced disease.

About 5% of patients presenting with chronic inflammatory back
pain have ankylosing spondylitis. If there is progression to ankylosis,
the inflammatory pain usually lessens but there is important
functional impairment

Ankylosis. The principal concern in patients with spondylitis is
progression towards ankylosis. The ankylosis is a consequence of
ossification of the ligaments and also, at the thoracic level, the
vertebrocostal and sternocostal joints. Physical examination reveals
impaired spinal mobility, with restricted flexion and extension of the

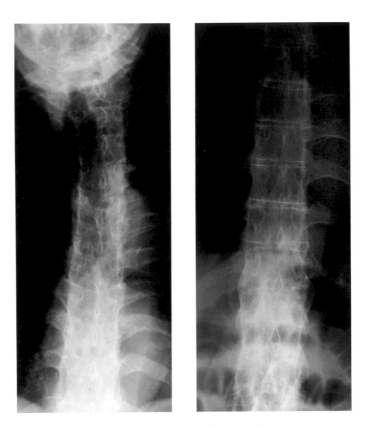

Figure 4.1 Anteroposterior view of ankylosed thoracic spine.

lumbar spine or limited chest expansion. The restriction in motion is not proportional to the degree of ankylosis, because of secondary muscle spasms.

In patients with restricted chest wall motion, airflow measurements are normal, but vital capacity is decreased and functional residual capacity is increased. Respiratory failure can occur in severe cases. However, ankylosis in the thoracic and lumbar spine (Figures 4.1 and 4.2) is not necessarily linked to severe physical limitations. By contrast, ankylosis at the cervical level has major physical consequences, as the patient is unable to turn the head.

Spine radiographs and CT scans show the following characteristic changes in the later stages of ankylosing spondylitis: squaring of the vertebrae, presence of syndesmophytes and, finally, the classic

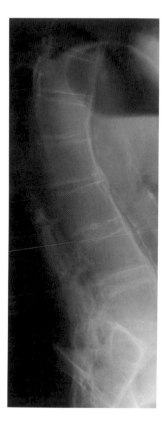

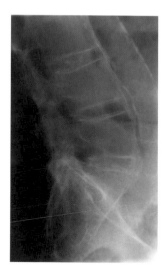

Figure 4.2 Lateral view of ankylosed lumbar spine.

ankylosed 'bamboo column' (Figure 4.3). Overall, computed tomography (CT) and plain radiography findings do not correlate well with disease activity.

Abnormal posture. Ankylosis of the spine in an abnormal position is more debilitating than ankylosis in an upright position, as it can have a major impact on functioning. The first sign of abnormal posture is loss of lumbar lordosis; this is followed by thoracic kyphosis and, in severe cases, by forward stooping of the neck (Figure 4.4). It is important to detect these abnormal features as early as possible, so that physiotherapy or other appropriate treatment can be considered.

Fracture. Spinal osteoporosis is often observed, especially in patients who have had severe ankylosing spondylitis for a long duration.

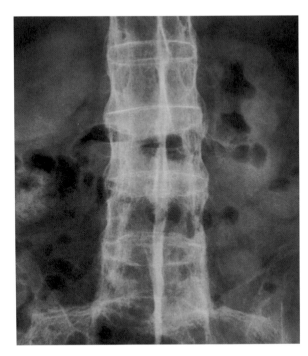

Figure 4.3
Anteroposterior view showing typical bamboo spine.

This contributes to the high prevalence of fractures; these fractures often occur after very minimal trauma to the rigid, ankylosed spine.

The spinal osteoporosis is partly due to the lack of mobility that is a consequence of ankylosis, but can also occur at a relatively early stage of the disease, perhaps as a result of proinflammatory cytokines. Assessment of biochemical markers of bone metabolism has shown that diminished bone formation and enhanced bone resorption are involved.

It is thought that osteoporotic fractures of the thoracic spine contribute to thoracic kyphosis and increased occiput-to-wall distance.

Sacroiliitis. Sacroiliac pain is typical of ankylosing spondylitis. Pain is described as occurring in the buttock, sometimes radiating to the posterior thigh. Pain in the sacroiliac joints is reproduced by applying direct pressure to the buttock over the site of the sacroiliac joint when the patient is lying prone with their legs extended. Other possible sacroiliac tests include: mobilizing the sacrum by direct pressure on the higher median part of the buttocks when the patient is lying prone;

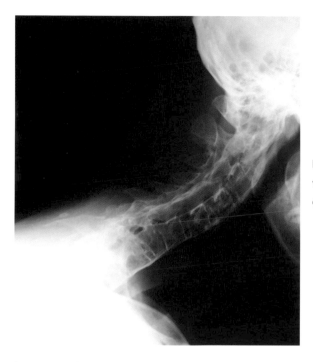

Figure 4.4 Lateral view of fused cervical spine.

hopping, which reactivates pain in the homolateral sacroiliac joint; and mobilization of the sacroiliac joint by bending the knee and hip to 90° and bringing the thigh into maximal abduction, with the patient supine. None of these tests is entirely specific or sensitive, hence most physicians practise several successively on the same patient before reaching a diagnosis of sacroiliac pain.

Sacroiliitis leads to functional impairment that affects walking. In addition, it often results in ankylosis; at this stage, the pain usually disappears.

The clinical diagnosis is supported by radiological evidence of sacroiliitis, which is still considered to be the radiographic hallmark of ankylosing spondylitis. Anteroposterior radiography of the pelvis is usually sufficient. However, unequivocal sacroiliac changes may not be evident on the radiographs until the disease has been present for many years. The earliest visible changes in the sacroiliac joints are blurring of the cortical margins of the subchondral bone, erosions and sclerosis. As erosion progresses, the joint space appears wider, then fibrous and bony ankylosis obliterates the joint. Joint changes usually become

37

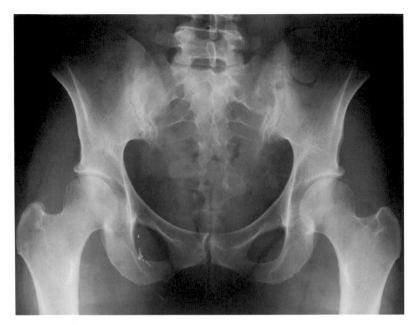

Figure 4.5 Grade III sacroiliitis.

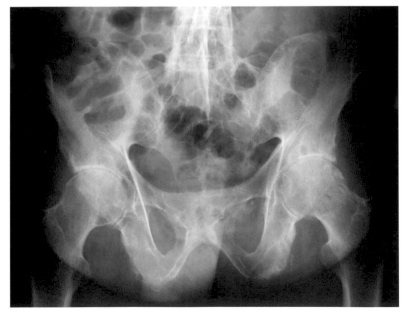

Figure 4.6 Grade IV sacroiliitis.

symmetrical during the course of the disease. The New York grading system for sacroiliac joint status is as follows: grade I, suspicious; grade II, evidence of erosion and sclerosis; grade III, erosions, sclerosis and early ankylosis; and grade IV, total ankylosis (Figures 4.5–4.6).

When clinical suspicion of early ankylosing spondylitis is high but standard radiography of the sacroiliac joints is normal or shows only equivocal changes, magnetic resonance imaging (MRI), especially with gadolinium enhancement, produces excellent radiation-free evidence of sacroiliitis and enthesitis. CT also can detect sacroiliitis.

A prospective evaluation has been carried out of the relative sensitivities of MRI, quantitative sacroiliac scintigraphy and plain radiography in detecting active sacroiliitis in 44 patients with clinical symptoms of inflammatory low back pain plus additional features of spondylarthropathy (mostly ankylosing spondylitis patients). MRI was found to be the most sensitive imaging technique (95% sensitivity, compared with 19% for plain radiography and 48% for quantitative sacroiliac scintigraphy). These findings indicate that MRI can detect an additional 76% of early sacroiliitis cases, compared with plain radiography. However, MRI and quantitative sacroiliac scintigraphy are expensive, can be difficult to obtain and are not always necessary; therefore, they are not routinely used.

Anterior chest wall and root joints. The term axial involvement is often considered to include inflammation of the anterior chest wall and root joints (shoulders and hips). Anterior chest wall pain occurs in about 15% of patients and is usually the result of sternoclavicular, manubriosternal or sternocostal arthritis. As stated above, this can lead to reduced chest expansion.

Arthritis occurs in the hips and shoulders in some patients, often early in the course of the disease. It is important to check for root joint involvement, as it can cause major disability. Hip involvement often leads to severe destruction, necessitating total hip replacement.

Peripheral arthritis
Peripheral arthritis is less common than axial involvement in ankylosing spondylitis. It is mostly oligoarticular, asymmetrical,

transient and migratory, with involvement of both small and large joints, predominantly of the lower limbs. A bilateral symmetrical polyarticular presentation is possible, which differs from rheumatoid arthritis in that the distal interphalangeal joints are often involved.

Inflammation of the peripheral joints may be apparent on physical examination. A typical feature is dactylitis ('sausage-like digit'), in which metacarpophalangeal and proximal interphalangeal arthritis is associated with tenosynovitis. Radiographs of the peripheral joints do not generally reveal erosions.

Enthesitis

Painful inflammation of entheses, the sites of bony insertion of ligaments and tendons, is a classic and frequent feature of ankylosing spondylitis. The most typical enthesitis is heel pain (posterior or inferior) related to inflammation of the Achilles tendon or the plantar fascia insertion. Pain appears in the morning, as soon as the patient sets his or her foot on the floor, then disappears after a few hours. Heel enthesitis is not painful during sleep. Other clinical indicators are tenderness of the iliac crest, anterior tibial tuberosity or anterior chest wall. Enthesitis is best visualized by ultrasonography and is not detected on radiographs.

Extra-articular features

All of the extra-articular features of spondylarthropathies may be seen in ankylosing spondylitis (see Chapter 1). Only the most common and/or severe features are detailed here.

Acute anterior uveitis. The most common extra-articular manifestation of ankylosing spondylitis is acute anterior uveitis, with 25–40% of patients experiencing one or more episodes. These episodes are more likely to occur in patients who are positive for HLA-B27.

It is important to detect and treat acute anterior uveitis rapidly, in order to protect the patient's eyesight. The condition typically presents with unilateral eye pain and redness, photophobia and increased lacrimation. Patients with these signs require urgent examination

by an ophthalmologist, who will provide specialized treatment
(e.g. retro-orbital injections of corticosteroids). Uveitis tends to
recur, sometimes in the contralateral eye.

Diarrhea. Inflammatory lesions in the gut are common in ankylosing
spondylitis and can result in diarrhea, which is usually accompanied
by blood and glairy mucus. Loss of weight is common. Inflammatory
bowel disease may or may not have already been diagnosed in
these patients.

Colonoscopic mucosal biopsy reveals that subclinical inflammatory
lesions are seen in 20–70% of patients with ankylosing spondylitis who
have no gastrointestinal symptoms or clinically obvious inflammatory
bowel disease. Follow-up studies of such patients indicate that 6% will
develop inflammatory bowel disease.

About 28–35% of patients with enteropathic arthritis have axial
disease: 10–20% have sacroiliitis alone, 7–12% have spondylitis and
10% have the classic features of ankylosing spondylitis. The axial
radiology is indistinguishable from that of uncomplicated ankylosing
spondylitis, although the frequency of asymmetrical sacroiliitis is
probably higher. The clinical picture may also be indistinguishable from
classic ankylosing spondylitis. The onset of axial involvement often
precedes that of bowel disease and axial symptoms do not fluctuate
with bowel disease activity.

Biological markers
Only 50–70% of patients with active disease exhibit biological markers
of inflammation, with elevated erythrocyte sedimentation rates (ESR)
and C-reactive-protein (CRP) levels; blood cell count is normal and
rheumatoid factor is negative. Mild normochromic normocytic anemia
may be detected. A raised alkaline phosphatase level may be present in
severe disease.

Prognosis
The course of ankylosing spondylitis varies considerably from patient to
patient and there may be spontaneous remissions or exacerbations,
particularly in the early stages. However, disease activity generally

persists for many decades, rarely entering long-term remission.

A large proportion of patients seen at an early stage will never develop spinal ankylosis. In those with ankylosis, there is an increasing degree of spinal ankylosis as the disease progresses. Loss of mobility often occurs in a kyphotic position, and dorsal ankylosis can result in loss of lung capacity. At an advanced stage, surgery is the only option. It is crucial to make every effort to prevent ankylosis in an abnormal position.

The most serious complication of ankylosing spondylitis is spinal fracture. Even minor trauma to the rigid, fragile spinal column can cause severe damage. The cervical spine is the most susceptible site; fracture in this region can result in neurological compression, and high morbidity and mortality.

Patients with a definite diagnosis of ankylosing spondylitis therefore face the probability of a lifetime of progressive structural deterioration and associated pain and functional disability, which will contribute to substantial socioeconomic loss and reduced quality of life.

Although the course of the disease cannot be predicted in the initial stages, research suggests that a predictable pattern emerges within the first 10 years. In a longitudinal study by Carette et al., the natural course of ankylosing spondylitis was examined over a 23-year period in 51 patients who had a mean disease duration of 38 years. Of the patients who had mild spinal restriction after 10 years, 74% did not progress to severe spinal involvement. In contrast, 81% of patients who had severe spinal involvement were severely affected within the first 10 years. There was sufficient disease progression to cause severe restriction of spinal mobility in about 40% of patients.

What are the predictive factors for long-term outcome? Amor et al. conducted a cohort study of 151 patients monitored by a single investigator over a period of at least 10 years. He found that hip arthritis was a strong predictive factor, being associated with a 23-fold increase in the risk of severe disease. Other factors that were associated with a high risk of severe disease are shown in Table 4.2. The absence of all of these factors during the first 2 years of the disease was predictive of a mild outcome (sensitivity 92.5%, specificity 78%).

TABLE 4.2

Factors predictive of severe disease and severe outcome

The following have been estimated by Amor to be predictive of
severe disease (specificity 97.5%, sensitivity 50%). The absence
of all of these factors during the first two years of the disease
was predictive of a mild outcome (sensitivity 92.5%,
specificity 78%)

- Hip involvement

or

- The presence of three of the following factors within 2 years
  of onset of ankylosing spondylitis
  - ESR > 30 mm in the first hour
  - unresponsiveness to non-steroidal anti-inflammatory drugs
  - limitation of lumbar spine movement
  - sausage-like finger or toe
  - oligoarthritis
  - onset at ≤ 16 years

There would appear to be some differences between the sexes in the
course of the disease. Many reports show that women have a later age
of onset, milder disease and greater extraspinal involvement.

It has also been shown that loss of function correlates significantly
with radiographic changes of ankylosing spondylitis in the spine, the
development of 'bamboo spine', and the occurrence of appendicular
(hip and shoulder) and peripheral arthritis.

Key points – clinical features

- Ankylosing spondylitis is 2–3 times more common in men than women.
- The initial symptom of ankylosing spondylitis is typically a dull inflammatory lower back pain of insidious onset, becoming persistent after a few months.
- Sacroiliac pain is typical of ankylosing spondylitis; pain is described as occurring in the buttock, sometimes radiating to the posterior thigh.
- The radiographic hallmarks of ankylosing spondylitis are signs of sacroiliitis, starting with blurring of the cortical margins of the subchondral bone, erosions and sclerosis. Later changes include joint space widening, followed by obliteration of the joint by fibrous and bony ankylosis.
- Arthritis of the peripheral joints is mostly oligoarticular, asymmetrical, transient and migratory, with involvement of both small and large joints, predominantly of the lower limbs.
- Painful inflammation of entheses, the sites of bony insertion of ligaments and tendons, is a classic feature of ankylosing spondylitis. The most typical enthesitis is inflammatory heel pain (posterior or inferior) responsible for 'first step' pain in the morning.
- Acute anterior uveitis is the most common extra-articular manifestation, with 25–40% of patients experiencing one or more episodes. It requires urgent referral to an ophthalmologist.
- The most serious complication of ankylosing spondylitis is functional impairment due to abnormal posture.
- A rare but severe complication is spinal fracture; even minor trauma to the rigid, fragile spinal column can cause major damage.

Key references

Amor B, Santos RS, Nahal R et al. Predictive factors of the long-term outcome of spondyloarthropathies. *J Rheumatol* 1994;21:1883–7.

Blackburn Jr WD , Alarcon GS, Ball GV. Evaluation of patients with back pain of suspected inflammatory nature. *Am J Med* 1988;85:766–70.

Blum U, Buitrago-Tellez C, Mundinger A et al. Magnetic resonance imaging (MRI) for detection of active sacroiliitis – a prospective study comparing conventional radiography, scintigraphy and contrast-enhanced MRI. *J Rheumatol* 1996;23: 2107–15.

Boonen A, van der Heijde D, Landewe R et al. Work status and productivity costs due to ankylosing spondylitis: comparison among three European countries. *Ann Rheum Dis* 2002;61:429–37.

Braun J, Bollow M, Sieper J. Radiologic diagnosis and pathology of the spondyloarthropathies. *Rheum Dis Clin North Am* 1998;24: 697–735

Burgos-Vargas R, Pacheco-Tena C, Vásquez-Mellado J. The juvenile-onset spondyloarthritides: rationale for clinical evaluation. *Best Pract Res Clin Rheumatol* 2002;16:551–72.

Carette S, Graham D, Little H et al. The natural disease course of ankylosing spondylitis. *Arthritis Rheum* 1983;26:186–90.

de Vlam K, de Vos M, Mielants H et al. Spondyloarthropathy is underestimated in inflammatory bowel disease; prevalence and HLA association. *J Rheumatol* 2000;27:2860–5.

Dougados M, van Der Linden S, Juhlin R et al. The European Spondyloarthropathy Study Group preliminary criteria for the classification of spondylarthropathy. *Arthritis Rheum* 1991;34:1218–27.

Keat A. Reiter's syndrome and reactive arthritis in perspective. *N Engl J Med* 1983;309:1606–15.

Khan MA. Ankylosing spondylitis: clinical features. In: Klippel JH, Dieppe PA, eds. *Rheumatology*. 2nd edn. London: Mosby-Wolfe, 1998:6.16.1–6.16.10.

Mitra D, Elvins DM, Speden DJ, Collins AJ. The prevalence of vertebral fractures in mild ankylosing spondylitis and their relationship to bone mineral density. *Rheumatology (Oxford)* 2000;39:87–9.

Spoorenberg A, van der Heijde D, de Klerk E et al. Relative value of erythrocyte sedimentation rate and C-reactive protein in assessment of disease activity in ankylosing spondylitis. *J Rheumatol* 1999;26:980–4.

van der Linden SJ, Valkenburg HA, Cats A. Evaluation of diagnostic criteria for ankylosing spondylitis. A proposal for modification of the New York criteria. *Arthritis Rheum* 1984;27:361–8.

Désirée van der Heijde

A careful history and clinical examination are of paramount importance in reaching a diagnosis of ankylosing spondylitis. Symptoms of inflammatory back pain and limitation of spine movement in all directions should lead the doctor to suspect ankylosing spondylitis. Laboratory values are of little assistance. Elevation of acute phase reactants such as ESR and CRP provides an additional argument for the diagnosis of ankylosing spondylitis, but there is no such elevation in the majority of patients. Hence, normal levels of acute phase reactants do not enable the disease to be excluded. Radiographs are often only helpful in later phases of the disease. The presence of a bilateral sacroiliitis makes the diagnosis certain. In early cases, active inflammation visible on an MRI of the sacroiliac joints is indicative of ankylosing spondylitis.

Validated instruments

Validated instruments are needed not only for assessing the efficacy of different treatments in clinical trials, but also for practical patient management. Such instruments help the physician to assess the prognosis, monitor the course of the disease and determine when to start treatment, as well as evaluating the efficacy of therapy. As Verna Wright wrote in 1983, 'clinicians may all too easily spend years writing "doing well" in the notes of a patient who has become progressively crippled before their eyes'.

The Assessment in Ankylosing Spondylitis (ASAS) Working Group, which comprises over 40 international experts in this field, has proposed three core sets of overlapping domains to facilitate evaluation of disease-controlling antirheumatic therapy (DCART) and symptom-modifying antirheumatic drugs (SMARD)/physical therapy, and to enhance record keeping (Figure 5.1). These core sets are suitable for use in clinical practice as well as in clinical trials.

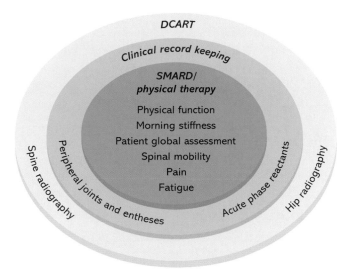

Figure 5.1 Three core sets of domains defined by the Assessment in Ankylosing Spondylitis (ASAS) Working Group to assist patient evaluation.

For each domain within the core sets, one or several instruments are available for assessing the patient. The core sets ensure that a minimum of required information is collected. Other data are likely to be needed, depending on the underlying research question or the particular clinical situation.

As shown in Figure 5.1, the domains of pain, patient global assessment of disease activity, morning stiffness, fatigue, spinal mobility and physical function are included in all of the core sets. The selected instruments per domain are presented in Table 5.1 and are discussed in more detail on pages 50–53.

Disease presentation

Four different features can be observed in patients with ankylosing spondylitis: axial involvement, peripheral joint involvement, enthesitis, and extra-articular signs and symptoms. Extra-articular features are not included in the core sets because they vary widely from patient to patient. In clinical practice, however, it is essential to check for the presence of these features, the most prevalent of

47

TABLE 5.1

Specific instruments for each domain in core sets for DCART, SMARD, physical therapy and clinical record keeping (from van der Heijde et al., 1999)

Domain	Instrument
Physical function	BASFI or Dougados Functional Index
Pain	VAS/NRS, last week, in spine, at night, due to ankylosing spondylitis *and* VAS/NRS, last week, in spine, due to ankylosing spondylitis
Spinal mobility	Chest expansion *and* modified Schober *and* occiput-to-wall distance *and* lateral spinal flexion or BASMI
Patient global assessment	VAS/NRS, last week
Morning stiffness	Duration of morning stiffness, in spine, last week
Fatigue	VAS/NRS, last week
Peripheral joints and entheses	Number of swollen joints (44-joint count) Validated enthesis indexes
Acute phase reactants	ESR
Spine radiographs	Anteroposterior + lateral lumbar *and* lateral cervical spine *and* X-ray pelvis (to visualize sacroiliac joint and hips)
Hip radiographs	As above

BASFI, Bath Ankylosing Spondylitis Functional Index; BASMI, Bath Ankylosing Spondylitis Metrology Index; CRP, C-reactive protein; DCART, disease-controlling antirheumatic therapy; ESR, erythrocyte sedimentation rate; NRS, numerical rating scale; SMARD, symptom-modifying antirheumatic drugs; VAS, visual analog scale
Included in core sets for DCART, SMARD/physical therapy, and clinical record keeping
Included in core sets for DCART and clinical record keeping
Included in core set for DCART

which are acute anterior uveitis, symptoms of inflammatory bowel disease and psoriasis. Early recognition of uveitis is particularly important, as immediate treatment is required to prevent the possibility of blindness.

Monitoring

A patient with isolated axial involvement can subsequently suffer from another clinical manifestation of ankylosing spondylitis. Patients should therefore be assessed systematically at each visit, whatever the initial clinical manifestation of the disease. The assessment can be performed using the various instruments that measure the different domains within the core sets. This will cover three of the four different groups of symptoms (i.e. axial involvement, peripheral joint involvement, enthesiopathy). It is also important for the physician to monitor extra-articular features.

Overall disease activity and functioning

An overall view of disease activity is given by the following domains: patient global assessment, pain, morning stiffness, fatigue and physical functioning. The physical functioning domain deserves special mention, as it is influenced both by disease activity and by disease severity.

Many instruments use a visual analog scale (VAS). This is a horizontal 10-cm line with two anchors: the left anchor represents the best situation (a score of 0) and right anchor represents the worst situation (a score of 10). Patients are asked to put a vertical mark at the position on the line that best represents their symptoms. The distance between the left anchor and the vertical mark is measured and recorded to one decimal point.

An alternative to a VAS is a numerical rating scale (NRS), which consists of a row of numbers from 0 to 10. The patient is asked to put a cross through the number that best represents their symptoms. The anchors (0 and 10) have the same meaning as on the VAS. An NRS has the following advantages over a VAS.

- It is better understood by patients.
- The results are immediately obvious without measuring.
- There are no extra sources of measurement error.
- It can be assessed by telephone.

It has been proven in several studies that there is no loss of information when using an NRS instead of a VAS. An example of a VAS and NRS for pain is presented in Figure 5.2. Use of an NRS can therefore be substituted for a VAS, if preferred.

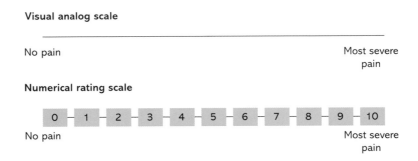

Figure 5.2 Example of a visual analog scale and a numerical rating scale.

Patient global assessment. The patient is asked to place a mark on a VAS or an NRS to represent their response to the question: 'How active was your spondylitis on average last week?'.

Pain. Patients are asked two questions about the pain experienced on average over the previous week. The first question is 'How much spine pain did you experience due to ankylosing spondylitis?', and the second is 'How much spine pain did you experience at night due to ankylosing spondylitis?' Patients indicate their response on a VAS or NRS.

Morning stiffness. The patient is asked: 'On average last week, for how long after you woke up did you experience stiffness in your spine?' This is recorded in minutes or on a VAS which has a maximum score of 2 hours.

Fatigue. One general question is asked about the average level of fatigue in the previous week: 'How would you describe the overall level of fatigue/tiredness you have experienced?' This, too, is answered on a VAS or NRS.

Physical function. Two indexes are available to assess functional capacity: the Bath Ankylosing Spondylitis Functional Index (BASFI) and the Dougados Functional Index. The BASFI consists of ten questions, answered on a VAS or NRS. The final score is the average of the scores on the ten questions, ranging from 0 (no limitation in function) to 10 (maximal limitation). The Dougados Functional Index has 20 questions, which are answered on a 3-point or 5-point verbal rating scale and summed to give a total score. The answers are scored 0, 1 and 2 or 0, 0.5, 1, 1.5 and 2, respectively, to ensure that the final score always falls in the range 0–40.

Both functional indexes have been shown to be valid and sensitive in differentiating between groups of patients with a different level and/or improvement in physical function. There seems to be little difference between the two instruments in their sensitivity to change.

Assessing spinal mobility

Assessment of the spinal mobility domain involves the use of all of the following four instruments.

Chest expansion. The patient is asked to rest their hands on or behind their head. The difference between maximal inspiration and expiration is then measured anteriorly at the fourth intercostal level (e.g. 4.4 cm). The better of two such measurements should be recorded.

Modified Schober test. The physician makes a mark on the patient's skin on the imaginary line between the two superior, posterior iliac spines. A second mark is then made 10 cm higher than the first mark. The patient is asked to bend forward as far as they can, and the distance between the two marks on the skin is measured. The increase in the distance is noted (e.g. if 13.4 cm is the distance measured between the lines when the patient is bent forward maximally, the recorded result would be 3.4 cm). The better of two tries is recorded.

Occiput-to-wall test. The patient stands with the heels and back against a wall, and with hips and knees as straight as possible. The chin should be held at the usual carrying level. The patient is asked to try as hard as they can to touch their head against the wall. The distance between the wall and the occiput is then measured in centimeters (e.g. 9.2 cm). The better of two tries is recorded.

Lateral spinal flexion. The patient stands as close to a wall as possible, with the shoulders level. The distance between the patient's middle fingertip and the floor is measured with a tape measure. The patient is asked to bend sideways as far as they can without bending the knees or lifting the heels, while attempting to keep the shoulders in the same plane. The new distance from middle fingertip to floor is measured and the difference between the two is noted. The better of two tries is recorded for full left and right lateral flexion. The mean of the left and right values gives the final result for lateral spinal flexion (expressed in centimeters to the nearest 0.1 cm).

Peripheral involvement

The 44-swollen-joint count should be assessed (Figure 5.3). Joints included are: acromioclavicular joints, humeroscapular joints,

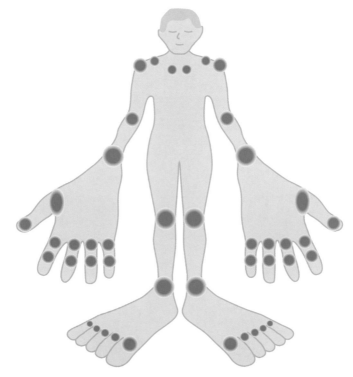

Figure 5.3 The 44-swollen-joint index

sternoclavicular joints, elbows, wrists, metacarpophalangeal
joints, proximal interphalangeal joints, knees, ankles and
metatarsophalangeal joints. In clinical practice, it is also important
to check for involvement of the manubriosternal and sternocostal
joints.

Enthesitis

A few validated enthesitis scores are available for clinical studies. In
clinical practice, painful sites should be examined. The plantar fascia
(heel pain) and the Achilles tendon are frequently involved. In fact, the
attachments of all tendons can be involved, but common sites are the
pelvis, symphysis pubis, thorax, spine and large joints.

Other assessments

Except for acute phase reactants, laboratory tests are of little value in
assessing patients with ankylosing spondylitis. The ESR after 1 hour
using the Westergren method and estimation of CRP levels can both be
useful for patient monitoring, but normal results do not exclude
inflammation. A significant proportion of patients with ankylosing
spondylitis do not have an elevated ESR or CRP.

Radiographs of the pelvis are important in making a diagnosis of
sacroiliitis. However, they provide little information for patient
monitoring. Radiographs of the spine show fast progression in a
minority of patients. It is not currently known how often radiographs
should be obtained in clinical practice, but the general expert opinion is
that more than once every two years is inappropriate.

For the ASAS core set, the instruments used in patient assessment
measure single variables only. In recent years, however, several
combined instruments have been developed, particularly by researchers
in Bath, UK. These pooled instruments assess various aspects of the
disease process. The Bath Ankylosing Spondylitis Disease Activity Index
(BASDAI) assesses signs and symptoms of disease activity such as
morning stiffness (duration and severity), several aspects of pain,
and fatigue. The Bath Ankylosing Spondylitis Metrology Index
(BASMI) combines information on various aspects of mobility
of the spine and hips.

Response criteria

The group results obtained from clinical trials using the various instruments for measuring core sets of domains are not always easy to translate to the individual patient level. Nevertheless, in clinical practice it is necessary for the physician to judge whether a treatment is effective for a particular patient. Therefore, criteria have been developed to assess the response that an individual with ankylosing spondylitis has to NSAID therapy. These ASAS response criteria are presented in Figure 5.4 and are based on the Dougados Functional Index or BASFI (the domain of function), morning stiffness (inflammation domain), patient global assessment (patient global domain), and overall pain (pain domain). In summary, three out of the four domains should each improve by at least 20% and a minimum of 10 units on a 100-point scale, and the remaining domain should show less than 20% worsening and less than a 10-unit deterioration. Using these criteria, a response rate of 49% has been observed in NSAID-treated patients in clinical trials, compared with 24% in patients receiving placebo.

In addition to the response criteria, partial remission criteria have been proposed to indicate the presence of very low levels of disease

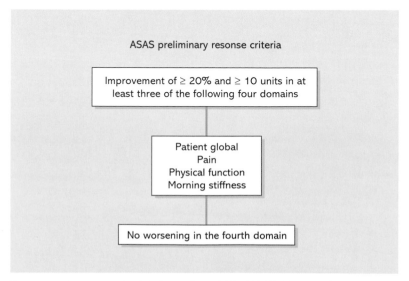

ASAS preliminary resonse criteria

Improvement of ≥ 20% and ≥ 10 units in at least three of the following four domains

Patient global
Pain
Physical function
Morning stiffness

No worsening in the fourth domain

Figure 5.4 Assessment in Ankylosing Spondylitis (ASAS) Working Group criteria for response to therapy.

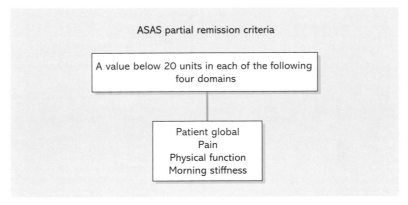

Figure 5.5 Assessment in Ankylosing Spondylitis (ASAS) Working Group criteria for partial remission.

activity (Figure 5.5). Partial remission is defined as a value below 20 (on a 100-point scale) in all four domains (function, inflammation, patient global and pain). By applying both the response and partial remission criteria to clinical trials, more information is available on the percentage of patients benefiting from therapy. The response and partial remission criteria can also be used in individual patients in clinical practice to assess the response to therapy and to assess the status of the patient.

Key points – assessment

- The Assessment in Ankylosing Spondylitis (ASAS) Working Group has proposed several core sets of overlapping domains to facilitate evaluation of therapy and enhance record keeping.
- The domains of pain, patient global assessment of disease activity, morning stiffness, fatigue, spinal mobility and physical function are included in all the core sets.
- Many instruments that assess these domains use a visual analog scale or a numerical rating scale.
- The ASAS Working Group has developed criteria for defining response to therapy and partial remission.
- These two sets of criteria are useful in clinical practice as well as in reporting clinical trial results.

Key references

van der Heijde D, Calin A, Dougados M et al. Selection of instruments in the core set for DC-ART, SMARD, physical therapy, and clinical record keeping in ankylosing spondylitis. Progress report of the ASAS Working Group. *J Rheumatol* 1999;26(4):951–4.

Anderson JJ, Baron G, van der Heijde D et al. Ankylosing spondylitis assessment group preliminary definition of short-term improvement in ankylosing spondylitis. *Arthritis Rheum* 2001;44(8):1876–86.

Dougados M, Gueguen A, Nakache JP et al. Evaluation of a functional index and an articular index in ankylosing spondylitis. *J Rheumatol* 1988;15:302–7.

Calin A, Garrett S, Whitelock H et al. A new approach to defining functional ability in ankylosing spondylitis: the development of the Bath Ankylosing Spondylitis Functional Index. *J Rheumatol* 1994;21:2281–5.

Astrid van Tubergen and Désirée van der Heijde

Physical therapy is often a necessary adjunct to drug therapy in ankylosing spondylitis and should therefore be considered in all patients. It may take the form of isometric or dynamic exercises, sporting activities or hydrotherapy (Table 6.1). The type of physical therapy selected will be influenced by the severity of the disease. The aim of physical therapy is to:

- maintain and improve mobility of the spine and peripheral joints
- strengthen the muscles of the trunk, legs, back and abdomen
- stretch the back and improve fitness through sporting activities
- relax the body and improve mobility by hydrotherapy.

Patients recently diagnosed with ankylosing spondylitis may first receive a course of supervised individualized therapy. After this, patients are expected to exercise daily without supervision. They are often advised to join weekly group physical therapy sessions, as this may help to maintain their motivation to exercise each day. In addition, many patients attend annual inpatient physiotherapy courses or spa therapy.

Patient education is a crucial aspect of successful management. As soon as the diagnosis of ankylosing spondylitis is made, patients must

TABLE 6.1

Forms of physical therapy in ankylosing spondylitis

- Supervised exercises
  - Individualized
  - Group physical therapy
- Unsupervised individualized exercises:
  - Disease-specific exercises
  - Recreational exercises
- Inpatient physiotherapy
- Spa therapy

be given clear explanations about the possible progression of their symptoms and other potential clinical features, as well as information about prognosis and treatment. Advising the patient about the possible occurrence of spinal ankylosis will enhance compliance with proposed treatments, especially physiotherapy

Exercise regimens

Supervised individualized exercises. Education plays a central role in supervised individualized exercises, which can be performed at a physiotherapy center or at home. The therapist advises the patient how to move and how to rest in a particular position. The aim is to teach the patient an individualized exercise program that they can subsequently continue at home, unsupervised, on a daily basis. The therapist also advises which sports are appropriate (e.g. badminton, volleyball, swimming) and which are not (e.g. horse-riding, cycling, football).

Unsupervised individualized exercises may consist of exercises learned in the supervised program, but may also include recreational exercises. These exercises should become part of the patient's daily routine.

Supervised group physical therapy. In practice, many patients find it difficult to comply with an individual daily exercise program. Supervised group physical therapy, usually consisting of physical exercises, sports and hydrotherapy, is offered mainly to motivate patients to continue exercising and to provide social contact with fellow sufferers. In addition, the supervising physiotherapist closely monitors the intensity of the exercises, in order to ensure that the patient will achieve the required improvement.

Inpatient physiotherapy. Recently diagnosed patients or those experiencing a flare of their disease are commonly offered inpatient physiotherapy at a specialized clinic. This consists of daily physical exercise and pool sessions for 2–4 weeks, complemented by education about the disease and information on patient societies.

Spa therapy. Courses of 2–4 weeks are offered, which may consist of balneotherapy (bathing in mineral water), hydrotherapy (immersion of all or parts of the body in water), massages, physical exercises, mud applications and relaxation sessions. In addition, attention is paid to health promotion through education and dietary regulation. Spa therapy can be provided on a group or individual basis.

Evidence for efficacy

A Cochrane review has recently assessed the available scientific evidence on the effectiveness of physiotherapeutic interventions in patients with ankylosing spondylitis. Randomized and quasi-randomized studies were included if at least one of the comparison groups received some type of physiotherapy. Of a total of 21 studies considered for inclusion, 18 were rejected due to inappropriate study design or because they were follow-up studies. Thus, a total of three randomized controlled trials met the inclusion criteria.

The reviewers concluded that there is a tendency toward positive short-term effects with physiotherapeutic intervention in ankylosing spondylitis. However, there is as yet insufficient evidence to make any firm recommendation for or against the use of physiotherapy in patients with ankylosing spondylitis. Study details and results are described below and shown in Table 6.2.

Supervised individualized exercises. In one randomized controlled trial, patients with ankylosing spondylitis were randomly allocated either to supervised individualized exercises and disease education at home (n = 26) or to no therapy (n = 27) for a period of 4 months. Compared with the control group, the intervention group showed a statistically significantly greater improvement in finger-to-floor distance (mean between-group improvement of 42%) and function (23%) at the end of the trial period.

Patients in the control group then received physiotherapy sessions at home for the next 4 months plus disease education. At the end of this open follow-up period, only function had changed significantly in both study groups, compared with results at 4 months.

TABLE 6.2

Effects of physical therapy on clinical outcome in ankylosing spondylitis

| | Domain | | | |
Therapy	Patient global	Physical function	Pain	Morning stiffness
Supervised individualized exercises	?	+	?	?
Unsupervised individualized exercises*	?	+	+	+
Group physical therapy	+	+	0	0
Inpatient physiotherapy	?	?	+	+
Spa therapy	+	+	+	0

+ = improvement; 0 = no change in comparison with control group; ? = not assessed
*Data from a longitudinal study only

Interestingly, the intervention group showed significantly greater improvement at 4 months than did the original control group at 8 months. This might be explained by the fact that the intervention group had received more therapy sessions in the first 4 months than did the original controls in the open follow-up period. This suggests that more frequent therapy given on a regular basis may be more effective.

Unsupervised individualized exercises. No randomized controlled trials have been conducted to investigate the effect of unsupervised exercises in ankylosing spondylitis. One longitudinal observational study described the effects of a median of 4.5 years of unsupervised exercises in 220 patients. A distinction was made between recreational exercise and back stretching or strengthening exercise. Health status improved most in patients involved in more than 200 minutes of recreational exercises each week or performing back exercises for at least 5 days per week.

Supervised group physical therapy. In one study, patients were randomly allocated to participate in weekly supervised group physical therapy in addition to daily unsupervised exercises at home (n = 68), or to a control group who were instructed only to exercise daily at home (unsupervised, n = 76). After 9 months, statistically significantly better results were reported in the intervention group for thoracolumbar flexion and extension (mean between-group improvement of 7%), physical fitness (5%) and global health (28%).

In a follow-on study, the original intervention group was randomized to continue receiving weekly supervised group physical therapy for another 9 months (n = 30) or to discontinue this therapy (n = 34; four patients lost to follow-up). Both of these groups were advised to continue exercising at home. After 9 months, there was a statistically significantly greater improvement in global health (28%) in the continuation group than in the discontinuation group. Function did not improve much in the continuation group (4%), but deteriorated significantly in the discontinuation group (–28%).

The time spent on exercises at home appeared to be significantly higher in the continuation group than in the discontinuation group. A possible explanation for this could be that the continuation group benefited from peer pressure and encouragement by the supervisor to perform the home exercises. The difference in the level of home exercising may account for part of the difference in outcomes in the study.

Inpatient physiotherapy. One study randomized patients with ankylosing spondylitis to one of the following three exercise regimens: 3 weeks of intensive inpatient physiotherapy (n = 15); twice-weekly hydrotherapy sessions with unsupervised individual exercises to be performed twice-daily at home over a 6-week period (n = 15); and unsupervised individual exercises at home (n = 14). All patients were advised to continue exercising at home after the treatment period.

Significant differences were found between the three groups immediately after the treatment period (i.e. at 6 weeks) in pain, stiffness and cervical rotation, with more improvement found in the two intervention groups than in the group doing unsupervised exercises at home. However, at 6 months no significant differences were found between the groups in any of the outcome measures.

Key points – physical therapy

- Physical therapy should be considered as part of the daily routine for patients with ankylosing spondylitis.
- Group physical therapy may enhance the effects of home exercising by providing a structured, supervised exercise program, which can increase the patient's motivation and hence compliance with unsupervised exercise.
- Inpatient physiotherapy and spa therapy can achieve rapid improvement, which may persist for several months.

Spa therapy. One randomized controlled trial has investigated the effect of spa therapy as an adjunct to standard treatment with drugs and weekly group physical therapy in patients with ankylosing spondylitis. Two groups of 40 patients each received treatment at two different spas (in Austria and the Netherlands) for 3 weeks, and subsequently followed weekly group physical therapy for 37 weeks. A control group (n = 40) stayed at home and participated in weekly group therapy for 40 weeks. After 3 weeks of spa therapy, both intervention groups showed significant improvement in functioning, patient global well-being and pain, compared with the control group at the same time-point. These benefits were maintained until 28 weeks after start of the intervention. The maximum between-group improvements were 24% for functioning, 30% for pain and 33% for global well-being. Spa therapy was also shown to be cost-effective (see page 30).

Choice of physical therapy modality

The available data indicate that physical exercises and spa therapy achieve positive effects in patients with ankylosing spondylitis. Each treatment modality has advantages and disadvantages. The advantages of group physical therapy over unsupervised therapy alone are mutual encouragement, increased motivation to carry out home exercises, exchange of experience, contact with fellow sufferers and personal feedback. Patients attending group physical exercises tend to spend more time on individual exercises than those who do not participate in the group programs.

A drawback is that group therapy is usually provided only once or twice a week. Patients may decide not to participate for practical, logistic reasons or simply because motivation and energy may not be optimal after working hours.

The advantages of inpatient physiotherapy or spa therapy are the intensive supervision, together with education and encouragement for the patients. There is also the possibility of achieving improvements within the short term. The main disadvantages are high cost and the difficulties that patients who are employed may encounter in being absent from work.

Future research is needed to determine the most effective physiotherapy modalities and applications for patients with ankylosing spondylitis. Meanwhile, patients should consider exercising as part of their daily routine. Depending on their personal needs, preferences, disease activity and severity, patients may opt for unsupervised exercise alone (either recreational or disease-specific exercises), or may also attend group physical therapy sessions. If necessary, they may undergo an inpatient physiotherapy course or engage in spa therapy. The treating physician should be convinced of the need for exercise treatment, and should then refer the patient to a physiotherapist. Inspired and motivated by the physiotherapist to follow the time-consuming exercise program, the patient may eventually benefit from a better disease outcome.

Key references

Bakker C, Hidding A, van der Linden S, van Doorslaer E. Cost effectiveness of group physical therapy compared to individualized therapy for ankylosing spondylitis. A randomized controlled trial. *J Rheumatol* 1994; 21:264–8.

Dagfinrud H, Hagen K. Physiotherapy interventions for ankylosing spondylitis (Cochrane review). *Cochrane Database of Systematic Reviews* 2001;4: Cd002822.

Helliwell PS, Abbott CA, Chamberlain MA. A randomised trial of three different physiotherapy regimens in ankylosing spondylitis. *Physiotherapy* 1996;82:85–90.

Hidding A, van der Linden S, Boers M et al. Is group physical therapy superior to individualized therapy in ankylosing spondylitis? A randomized controlled trial. *Arthritis Care Res* 1993;6:117–25.

Hidding A, van der Linden S, Gielen X et al. Continuation of group physical therapy is necessary in ankylosing spondylitis: results of a randomized controlled trial. *Arthritis Care Res* 1994;7:90–6.

Kraag G, Stokes B, Groh J et al. The effects of comprehensive home physiotherapy and supervision on patients with ankylosing spondylitis – a randomized controlled trial. *J Rheumatol* 1990;17:228–33.

Kraag G, Stokes B, Groh J et al. The effects of comprehensive home physiotherapy and supervision on patients with ankylosing spondylitis – an 8-month follow-up. *J Rheumatol* 1994;21:261–3.

van Tubergen A, Landewé R, van der Heijde D et al. Combined spa-exercise therapy is effective in patients with ankylosing spondylitis: a randomized controlled trial. *Arthritis Rheum* 2001;45:430–8.

van Tubergen A, Boonen A, Landewé R et al. Cost-effectiveness of combined spa-exercise therapy in ankylosing spondylitis: a randomized controlled trial. *Arthritis Rheum* 2002; 47:459–67.

Uhrin Z, Kuzis S, Ward MM. Exercise and changes in health status in patients with ankylosing spondylitis. *Arch Int Med* 2000; 160:2969–75.

7 Non-steroidal anti-inflammatory drug therapy

Corinne Miceli-Richard and Maxime Dougados

Non-steroidal anti-inflammatory drugs (NSAIDs) are the first-line treatment for those with ankylosing spondylitis and, to a large extent, for any other patients with painful clinical manifestations of arthritis or enthesitis that fall within the category of spondylarthropathy. Diagnosis and prognosis in ankylosing spondylitis depend on the patient's response to NSAIDs. Whether or nor biotherapies are indicated also depends on the response to NSAIDs. Recently defined criteria for disease response and remission following NSAID therapy represent the first step towards well-defined guidelines for short-term and long-term management of ankylosing spondylitis with these drugs.

History of NSAIDs

Before the development of anti-inflammatory drugs, the therapeutic options for ankylosing spondylitis were extremely limited. Considerable advances have been made over the past 60 years, which have maintained the efficacy of NSAIDs while reducing adverse events. This has provided rheumatologists with an effective first-line treatment for ankylosing spondylitis and many other inflammatory conditions.

Phenylbutazone was the first drug known as an NSAID. It was discovered in 1946 and introduced into clinical practice 3 years later, after World War 2. Phenylbutazone was very effective in ankylosing spondylitis but was associated with serious adverse events, notably aplastic anemia. This motivated the development of a second generation of NSAIDs with better safety profiles.

Indometacin was introduced in 1963. This drug had a similar efficacy to phenylbutazone and was also associated with serious adverse events, such as gastrointestinal bleeding, ulceration and perforation. Since that time, the pharmaceutical industry has been committed to developing well-tolerated drugs with potent anti-inflammatory effects. Various NSAIDs have been proposed for treating the symptoms of ankylosing spondylitis, including ibuprofen, ketoprofen, naproxen (all 1975), diclofenac (1976) and piroxicam (1981). Clinical trials have demonstrated that these drugs have comparable efficacy in patients with ankylosing spondylitis, with good tolerance profiles. The recently developed specific cyclo-oxygenase 2 inhibitors (COX-2 inhibitors) have been shown to be as effective as traditional NSAIDs in ankylosing spondylitis, and are particularly recommended for patients with peptic ulcer disease.

Phenylbutazone is now restricted to NSAID-refractory patients with severe disease. It should be prescribed only by experienced rheumatologists and with close hematologic monitoring, so that any bone marrow suppression may be detected early.

NSAIDs as a diagnostic tool

NSAIDs have a rapid and remarkable symptomatic effect in patients with ankylosing spondylitis, leading to the proposal that this is used as a diagnostic criterion. It is used in the Amor classification, which includes 12 items that each count for 1–3 points (see Chapter 1). A minimum of 6 points is necessary to classify a patient as suffering from spondylarthropathy. Item 12 in the Amor classification relates to NSAIDs efficacy: 'clear-cut improvement within 48 hours after NSAID intake or rapid relapse of pain after their discontinuation'. It carries a value of 2 points in this classification, illustrating the importance of the response to NSAIDs in reaching a diagnosis.

A multicenter cross-sectional study conducted in 741 patients complaining of back pain (69 with ankylosing spondylitis and 672 controls) estimated that the positive predictive value of NSAID efficacy was 34% and the negative predictive value was 97%. In this particular population of patients, the probability of ankylosing spondylitis was therefore very low (3%) if NSAIDs were ineffective.

Disease management

Overall, NSAIDs are effective in alleviating every painful manifestation of ankylosing spondylitis. However, the efficacy varies according to disease location, with axial involvement and/or enthesitis being classically more sensitive to NSAIDs, compared with peripheral arthritis. NSAIDs reduce pain, improve function and help to maintain normal mobility.

A long-acting NSAID taken at bedtime is recommended to manage the inflammatory and painful phases of the disease that occur at night. A morning dose of a short-acting NSAID may also be necessary. The response to specific NSAIDs often differs markedly between patients, so several drugs may need to be tried before an effective option is identified for a particular patient. The drug must be used at an appropriate dose before being considered inefficient; high doses are sometimes required in severe cases.

It remains unresolved whether an effective NSAID should be administered continuously or on demand. Continuous administration may facilitate concomitant physical therapy, but may also increase the risk of toxicity, particularly gastrointestinal adverse events. In clinical practice, the current view is to restrict NSAID administration to the active phase of the disease. If there is disease remission, a 'therapeutic window' can distinguish between an NSAID-related improvement (requiring continuation of drug treatment) and the onset of a non-active phase of the disease (that does not justify continued treatment). If a flare-up occurs when NSAIDs are discontinued, the drug should be reintroduced.

Structural effect

The correlation between short-term improvement and long-term outcome is still under debate. Forty years ago, ankylosing spondylitis patients often had a poor functional outcome. Since then, the functional prognosis has improved and it has been suggested that this is due to the use of NSAIDs as first-line symptomatic treatment. There is, as yet, no radiological evidence that NSAIDs have a significant effect on the structural progression of the disease. However, a placebo-controlled study comparing various NSAIDs (piroxicam or high- or low-dose meloxicam) showed improvement in chest expansion and CRP levels after 1 year of treatment, but not after 6 months. This supports a disease-controlling effect of NSAIDs with long-term use. Further long-term studies of NSAIDs are necessary to confirm this hypothesis. If true, this would have a considerable impact on rheumatological practice.

Short-term improvement criteria

The ASAS Working Group, created in 1995, proposed a standardized means of assessing clinical and laboratory outcome variables in ankylosing spondylitis. This group works in close cooperation with the Outcome Measures in Rheumatoid Arthritis Clinical Trials (OMERACT) Group (whose primary interest is the design of clinical studies in rheumatology) and international organizations such as the International League Against Rheumatism (ILAR) and the World Health Organization (WHO).

Five important domains were proposed by ASAS for the assessment of patients with ankylosing spondylitis: physical function, pain, spinal mobility, spinal stiffness/inflammation and patient's global assessment (fatigue has been added recently). Standard relevant criteria for response and remission (see Chapter 5) were then developed within four of these domains (physical function, pain, spinal inflammation/stiffness and patient's global assessment), to allow better evaluation of the efficacy of short-acting drugs in ankylosing spondylitis. Both sets of criteria were based on data from placebo-controlled trials that evaluated NSAIDs. The investigators did not include criteria for the spinal mobility measures because the results of short-term trials showed that currently available drugs did not improve spinal mobility.

Using the standard criteria, the expected response rates for patients who are naïve to treatment are 24% for placebo and 49% for NSAID treatment. The expected remission rate is 3% with placebo and 11% with NSAIDs. This composite set of responder criteria dramatically aids communication between physicians in daily practice, and also facilitates comparisons between clinical trial results, through homogenous presentation of data.

Discriminating between NSAIDs

It is usually easy to detect short-term efficacy of an NSAID relative to placebo in patients with ankylosing spondylitis, because there is only a minor placebo effect on function. For example, a recent double-blind, placebo-controlled study compared celecoxib (a COX-2 specific inhibitor), ketoprofen and placebo. Significant functional improvement was noted for both NSAID treatments ($p = 0.05$ and $p = 0.0006$, respectively), with no significant effect in the placebo group.

It is much more difficult, however, to establish a dose effect or a difference in efficacy between two or more NSAIDs. The short duration of trials, often no more than a few weeks, appears insufficient to identify the optimal dose regimen of the tested drugs.

In another placebo-controlled study, there was a 12-month double-blind extension to the original 6-week trial period in order to define the optimum study duration for identifying efficacy (and tolerance) of an active NSAID in ankylosing spondylitis. The investigators compared placebo (n = 121) with the following NSAIDs: piroxicam 20 mg/day (n = 108), meloxicam 15 mg/day (n = 120) and meloxicam 22.5 mg/day (n = 124). Life-table analysis of the patients still taking the study drug over time was used as it was considered to be more sensitive in detecting efficacy than the more common method of mean changes or percentage of responders. Each of the active drugs compared favorably with placebo, and there was a statistically significant difference in efficacy in favor of meloxicam 22.5 mg ($p < 0.05$), compared with either piroxicam 20 mg or meloxicam 15 mg. This difference in efficacy was not detected in the original 6-week study, suggesting that a 52-week study period is more appropriate for identifying such a difference between two active NSAIDs or between two different doses of a given NSAID.

Patients refractory to NSAIDs

Other treatments should be considered when NSAID therapy is ineffective, including anti-TNFα therapy. It would be useful in clinical practice to have a precise definition of the characteristics of a patient who is refractory to NSAID therapy. How many NSAIDs must be tested before a patient is considered refractory to NSAID therapy? In addition, for each NSAID, what dosage and duration of intake are required before the patient is deemed refractory to that particular NSAID? There is as yet no consensus on the definition of refractoriness to NSAID therapy.

A questionnaire was submitted to 28 international ankylosing spondylitis experts during the International Workshop on New

Treatment Strategies in Ankylosing Spondylitis (Berlin, January 2002). NSAID treatment failure was defined as failure of more than two NSAIDs by 54% of the experts, and as failure of more than three NSAIDs by 23%. Most experts (73%) thought that NSAID treatment should have been tried at the maximum recommended dose before it could be regarded as having failed.

Key points – non-steroidal anti-inflammatory drug therapy

- Phenylbutazone was the first anti-inflammatory drug to be discovered and was introduced into clinical practice in 1949.
- NSAID treatment results in improvement in pain and function, and contributes to maintenance of normal mobility.
- The effects of NSAID therapy on long-term outcome are unknown.
- Patients who are refractory to NSAIDs are potential candidates for biotherapies, such as anti-TNFα.

Key references

Amor B, Dougados M, Mijiyawa M. Critères de classification des spondylarthropathies. *Rev Rhum* 1990;57:85–9.

Anderson J, Baron G, van der Heijde D et al. Ankylosing Spondylitis Assessment Group preliminary definition of short-term improvement. *Arthritis Rheum* 2001;44:1876–86.

Dougados M, Behier JM, Jolchine I et al. Efficacy of celecoxib, a cyclooxygenase-2-specific inhibitor, in the treatment of ankylosing spondylitis: a six-week controlled study with comparison against placebo and against a conventional non-steroidal anti-inflammatory drug. *Arthritis Rheum* 2001;44:180–5.

Dougados M, Gueguen A, Nakache JP et al. Ankylosing spondylitis: what is the optimum duration of a clinical study? A one year versus a 6 weeks non-steroidal anti-inflammatory drug trial. *Rheumatology* 1999;38:235–44.

Dougados M, Nguyen M, Caporal R et al. Ximoprofen in ankylosing spondylitis: a double blind placebo controlled dose ranging study. *Scand J Rheumatol* 1994;23:243–8.

van der Heijde D, Bellamy N, Calin A et al. Preliminary core sets for endpoints in ankylosing spondylitis. Assessment in Ankylosing Spondylitis Working Group. *J Rheumatol* 1997;24:2225–9.

van der Heijde D, Calin A, Dougados M et al. Selection of instruments in the core set for DC-ART, SMARD, physical therapy and clinical record-keeping in ankylosing spondylitis. Progress report of the ASAS Working Group. *J Rheumatol* 1999;26:951–4.

Désirée van der Heijde

Although NSAIDs remain the cornerstone of treatment for ankylosing spondylitis, they may be ineffective or poorly tolerated in some patients. This has led to the so-called disease-modifying antirheumatic drugs (DMARDs), which are effective in rheumatoid arthritis, being tested in patients with ankylosing spondylitis.

The ASAS Working Group has proposed that the term disease-controlling antirheumatic therapy (DCART) be used to describe agents that achieve all of the following:

- reduced signs and symptoms
- improved or sustained physical function
- prevention or a significant decrease in the rate of progression of structural damage.

No therapy has yet proven to be efficacious in all three of these domains. Traditional DMARDs such as sulfasalazine and methotrexate, which are efficacious in rheumatoid arthritis, are of little value in ankylosing spondylitis. It is possible that drugs that have been less studied in rheumatoid arthritis, such as bisphosphonates and thalidomide, might suppress disease activity in patients with ankylosing spondylitis. However, data on most drugs are currently limited, as placebo-controlled studies with sufficient numbers of patients are often lacking. Moreover, there is often limited diagnostic information available about the patients included in the studies. Interpretation of data would be enhanced if it were known whether the disease was purely axial or predominantly peripheral.

The various treatment options for patients who respond poorly to or who are intolerant of NSAID therapy are discussed below. One recently available option is the group of drugs known as TNFα blocking agents, which appear very effective in treating ankylosing spondylitis.

Sulfasalazine

Sulfasalazine is the most widely studied conventional second-line agent in ankylosing spondylitis, with more than 10 double-blind trials reported. However, its efficacy remains unclear. A meta-analysis based on five smaller studies found that sulfasalazine had a limited efficacy in alleviating clinical symptoms. This could not be confirmed, however, in two large placebo-controlled studies. One of these larger studies showed no benefit in patients with pure axial disease, but there was a treatment effect in patients with mainly peripheral arthritis. In summary, if sulfasalazine has a positive effect on ankylosing spondylitis, it may be limited to the group of patients who have predominantly peripheral involvement.

The recommended dose of sulfasalazine is 2–3 g/day. Adverse effects are often seen and may sometimes limit the use of this drug. However, most side effects are mild and reversible on drug withdrawal. Common adverse effects of sulfasalazine include malaise, nausea, headache and dizziness. Hepatotoxicity and hematologic abnormalities, mainly neutropenia, are also encountered. Hypersensitivity reactions occur rarely. Reduced male fertility is a frequent adverse effect, but fertility recovers after discontinuation of the drug and there is no known teratogenecity.

Methotrexate

Methotrexate is highly efficacious in treating rheumatoid arthritis, particularly when used in doses up to 20–25 mg/week. Unfortunately, no placebo-controlled studies have been undertaken in patients with ankylosing spondylitis. All available data are from small open studies with relatively low doses of methotrexate (7.5–15 mg/week). These data are of limited value, and do not support the use of methotrexate in the treatment of ankylosing spondylitis.

Gold, antimalarials and azathioprine

There are a large number of case reports of treatment with gold and antimalarials, but no evidence to show that these agents are more effective than placebo in the treatment of ankylosing spondylitis. A double-blind study of azathioprine showed both a low response rate and a high withrawal rate due to adverse effects. Thus, none of these drugs is recommended in the treatment of patients with ankylosing spondylitis.

Corticosteroids

Corticosteroids have been used in ankylosing spondylitis patients in several ways:

- oral low-dose treatment
- intravenous pulse therapy
- intra-articular injections.

There is no evidence that oral low-dose corticosteroid treatment is efficacious in ankylosing spondylitis. One study reported that high-dose intravenous therapy (1000 mg methylprednisolone on 3 consecutive days) reduced clinical disease activity, but another study found that a high-dose regimen (1000 mg on 3 consecutive days) was not significantly more efficacious than a lower dose regimen (375 mg on 3 consecutive days). Given the limited data, no meaningful conclusion can be drawn regarding the role of either oral or intravenous corticosteroids in the treatment in ankylosing spondylitis.

Intra-articular injection of corticosteroids often leads to an immediate relief of symptoms in peripheral arthritis. Due to the anatomy of the sacroiliac joints, it is more difficult to give an intra-articular injection in cases of active sacroiliitis, so this treatment option is not common in clinical practice. However, several open studies and one controlled study have evaluated injection of the sacroiliac joints under CT or MRI guidance. The results showed that this was a safe and effective procedure, in expert hands, for reducing inflammatory back pain.

Bisphosphonates

Pamidronate is the most potent bisphosphonate available for intravenous use. Its efficacy in suppressing inflammation in ankylosing spondylitis has mainly been tested in patients with refractory disease. Several dose regimens have been investigated, most involving either monthly intravenous injections of 30–60 mg or a schedule of infusions on days 1, 2, 14, 28 and 56. Significant improvements in many clinical disease activity variables, including axial and peripheral involvement, have been reported in the various studies.

Adverse effects of pamidronate include transient asymptomatic hypocalcemia, transient lymphopenia, bone pain, and infusion reactions (including myalgia, arthralgia and pyrexia). Infusion reactions are present in a high percentage of patients after the first infusion, but usually not after subsequent infusions. The reactions are generally mild and last for 24–48 hours.

Further research is warranted into the optimal dose regimen of pamidronate, the efficacy of oral bisphosphonates and the effects on structural damage. Meanwhile, pamidronate is an option for patients with refractory ankylosing spondylitis.

Thalidomide

Based on its pharmacological properties, thalidomide is considered to be a TNFα blocking agent.

Thalidomide gained a bad reputation in the early 1960s because it is highly teratogenic and is also associated with peripheral neuropathies. More recently, it has been investigated under tightly controlled conditions for the treatment of severe, refractory ankylosing spondylitis. Several small open uncontrolled studies have been carried out using doses in the range of 100–300 mg/day and follow-up periods of 3–12 months. These studies show clinical improvement in a large proportion of patients, with a wide range of premature discontinuation rates in the various studies. In general, the tolerability of the drug was poor to moderate at the optimal dose. A controlled trial is needed before it can be decided whether thalidomide has a place in the treatment of ankylosing spondylitis.

TNFα blocking agents

TNFα is a cytokine that has been shown to mediate inflammatory and regulatory activities in immune-mediated diseases, including ankylosing spondylitis. Biological agents that block TNFα are among the new therapeutic options currently being investigated in ankylosing spondylitis.

The two major TNFα blocking agents that have demonstrated efficacy in the treatment of ankylosing spondylitis are the chimeric monoclonal IgG1 antibody infliximab, and the 75 kDa IgG1 receptor fusion protein etanercept. In contrast to conventional treatments, these agents target the specific inflammatory processes associated with ankylosing spondylitis. There have been many open-label studies and a few placebo-controlled double-blind studies of infliximab and etanercept. Infliximab is usually given as an infusion of 5 mg/kg body weight at weeks 0, 2 and 6, and thereafter at 6-weekly intervals; etanercept is given as a twice-weekly subcutaneous 25 mg injection.

All studies have shown major improvements in clinical and functional assessments in most patients, based on the ASAS20 response or improvement in BASDAI or BASFI. Furthermore, many patients show greater improvements, as assessed by an ASAS50 response (which differs from the ASAS20 response only in requiring an improvement of 50% and 20 units in at least three domains) or a 50% reduction in BASDAI.

For example, in a trial comparing infliximab with placebo, almost 50% of patients treated with infliximab showed an ASAS50 response, compared with 6% in the placebo group. In addition, 21% fulfilled the ASAS criteria for partial remission, compared with 0% in the placebo group. In a controlled trial of etanercept, over 70% of patients on active treatment showed a clinical response, compared with 30% in the placebo group. The controlled trials were all of short duration, but in the open follow-up period the effects were maintained. Moreover, the first effects were seen as early 2 weeks after start of therapy. In addition to the effects on signs, symptoms and physical function, there was also reduced inflammation as assessed by MRI of the spine and sacroiliac joints.

The effect of TNFα blocking agents on the progression of structural damage is currently under investigation. Given the good clinical effect and the reduction in spinal inflammation on MRI, there are high expectations that these investigations will reveal a significant reduction in the progression of structural damage.

Areas of concern. The relatively short experience with TNFα blockers means that the full spectrum and frequency of adverse events is not yet established. Based on the mechanism of action, the results of clinical trials and postmarketing data (mainly when prescribed for other indications, such as rheumatoid arthritis, psoriatic arthritis and

Crohn's disease), there are several areas of concern. The two most important are:

- infections, including sepsis and tuberculosis
- malignancy, including lymphoma.

A large number of cases of tuberculosis have been reported in patients using TNFα blocking agents. Therefore, it is advisable to check patients for the presence of latent tuberculosis (using the local guidelines) before initiating TNFα blocking agents. Since the adoption of this measure, there has been a dramatic drop in the incidence of tuberculosis. Nevertheless, patients still need to be followed carefully because infections, including sepsis, may have an atypical course.

An increase in malignancies can be expected among patients receiving TNFα blocking agents. This is based mainly on theoretical grounds, because there are as yet no data showing an increased incidence of malignancy in those receiving TNFα blocking therapy.

Other frequent, but usually mild, adverse events are infusion reactions with infliximab and injection site reactions with etanercept.

ASAS recommendations. Overall, the risks associated with TNFα blocking agents appear to be small. Given the dramatic efficacy, there is a favorable risk:benefit ratio. Recently, the ASAS Working Group achieved international consensus on the use of TNFα blocking agents in ankylosing spondylitis. They recommend that TNFα blocking agents should be prescribed only by doctors who are specialists in the treatment of ankylosing spondylitis and also in the use of these specific agents. In addition, patients should normally fulfil the modified New York criteria for definite ankylosing spondylitis and have active disease for at least 4 weeks before treatment with TNFα blocking agents is initiated. Active disease is defined as a BASDAI score of at least 4 (on a 10-point scale) plus the opinion of an expert that treatment is indicated. All patients must have an adequate trial of at least two NSAIDs. An adequate trial is defined as treatment for at least 3 months at the maximal recommended or tolerated anti-inflammatory dose, unless contraindicated. Treatment for less than 3 months is acceptable when treatment was withdrawn because of intolerance or toxicity or contraindications. Patients with symptomatic peripheral arthritis

---

Key points – disease-controlling antirheumatic therapy

- As yet, no treatment fulfils all three requirements for disease-controlling antirheumatic therapy.
- Conventional disease-modifying antirheumatic drugs used in rheumatoid arthritis are not effective in ankylosing spondylitis.
- Only sulfasalazine shows some efficacy in patients with peripheral involvement.
- Pamidronate can be tried in patients with severe refractory ankylosing spondylitis.
- Tumor necrosis factor α (TNFα) blocking agents (infliximab and etanercept) appear to be very effective in the treatment of both axial and peripheral manifestations of ankylosing spondylitis.
- Guidelines are available on the initiation of TNFα blocking agents and for monitoring the efficacy of this treatment.

---

must have had an adequate therapeutic trial of NSAIDs and also sulfasalazine. Those with oligoarticular involvement should usually also have failed local steroid injections.

Sulfasalazine should be tried for at least 4 months at the standard target dose or the maximally tolerated dose, unless contraindicated. Treatment for less than 4 months is acceptable if the drug was withdrawn because of intolerance, toxicity or contraindications. Patients with symptomatic enthesitis must have an adequate therapeutic trial of at least two local steroid injections, unless contraindicated.

Treatment efficacy should be evaluated 6–12 weeks after the start of treatment with TNFα blocking agents. A sufficient response to warrant continuation of therapy has been defined as an improvement of 50% in BASDAI or an absolute improvement of 2 (on a 10-point scale) together with the expert opinion that therapy should be continued.

The implications of these guidelines will be investigated in the near future.

Key references

Braun J, Breban M, Maksymowych W. Therapy for ankylosing spondylitis: new treatment modalities. *Best Pract Res Clin Rheumatol* 2002;16:631–52.

Braun J, Pham T, Sieper J et al. for the ASAS Working Group. International ASAS consensus statement for the use of biologic agents in patients with ankylosing spondylitis. *Ann Rheum Dis* 2003;62:817–24.

Braun J, Sieper J, Breban M et al. Anti-tumour necrosis factor alpha therapy for ankylosing spondylitis: international experience. *Ann Rheum Dis* 2002;61(suppl 3):iii51–60.

Dougados M, Dijkmans B, Khan M et al. Conventional treatments for ankylosing spondylitis. *Ann Rheum Dis* 2002;61(suppl 3):iii40–50.

Dougados M, van der Linden S, Leirisalo-Repo M et al. Sulfasalazine in the treatment of spondylarthropathy. A randomized, multicenter, double-blind, placebo-controlled study. *Arthritis Rheum* 1995;38:618–27.

Haibel H, Braun J, Maksymowych W. Bisphosphonates – targeting bone in the treatment of spondylarthritis. *Clin Exp Rheumatol* 2002;28(suppl): S162–6.

Huang F, Wei J, Breban M. Thalidomide in ankylosing spondylitis. *Clin Exp Rheumatol* 2002;28(suppl):S158–61.

Maksymowych W, Breban M, Braun J. Ankylosing spondylitis and current disease-controlling agents: do they work? *Best Pract Res Clin Rheumatol* 2002;16:619–30.

van der Horst-Bruinsma I, Clegg D, Dijkmans B. Treatment of ankylosing spondylitis with disease modifying antirheumatic drugs. *Clin Exp Rheumatol* 2002;28(suppl):S67–70.

9 Future trends

Désirée van der Heijde and Maxime Dougados

Biological therapy

In the near future, more information will become available about the effectiveness of biological therapy, particularly anti-TNFα therapy. Data will be reported from longer-term follow-up studies of agents already approved for treating for ankylosing spondylitis, as well as from trials of other compounds. In addition, the effects that different agents have in various domains will be further elucidated. For example, it has been suggested that anti-TNFα therapy may inhibit the progression of structural damage to the spine. Data will be collected that will prove or refute this suggestion. Spinal mobility is another important domain in which the effects of anti-TNFα therapy will become clearer with time.

As experience of anti-TNFα therapy in clinical practice increases, involving larger numbers of patients with more heterogeneous disease than in clinical trials, it will become apparent which individuals benefit most from treatment. This will make it clearer who should be treated with this therapy. Wider use will also give better insight into the risks of treatment. Given the cost of anti-TNFα therapy, there is likely to be major interest in the socioeconomic consequences of the disease and the short- and long-term cost-effectiveness of these biological agents.

Diagnosis

Increased efforts will be made to facilitate early diagnosis of ankylosing spondylitis. At present, there is a delay of about 10 years between onset of the first symptoms and diagnosis. One prerequisite for earlier diagnosis is better education of healthcare professionals.

Improved assessment techniques may enable the diagnosis to be made earlier, perhaps using a different combination of disease features. Use of MRI, for example, may allow inflammation to be detected before permanent damage is visible on radiographs (which could take several years).

It will be even more important to diagnose the disease promptly if anti-TNFα therapy is shown to improve outcome, so that treatment can be initiated before permanent damage occurs.

Prognosis

It is also useful to be able to identify patients who have a poor prognosis. These individuals may have a high risk of significant functional impairment or work disability, or be likely to need hip replacement surgery. Such patients are high-priority candidates for receiving the most effective treatment strategies available. In addition, it is helpful to know which patients are likely to respond best to certain treatments, as this will enable clinicians to optimize treatment strategies.

Imaging

Sensitive scoring methods for structural damage on plain films will give a better insight into the course of the disease; they can also be used to establish the effectiveness of treatment in preventing or reducing structural damage. Improved scoring techniques will also help to clarify the relationship between spinal mobility and radiographic evidence of damage, as well as disease activity and the progression of structural damage. Combined with information on bone and cartilage markers, this may elucidate the pathogenesis of the disease.

Furthermore, by combining information from MRI and plain radiography, it should be possible to differentiate inflammatory changes from structural damage. This, too, could lead to new insights into the pathogenesis of ankylosing spondylitis.

In addition, ultrasound may provide more information about the occurrence, course and treatment of enthesitis in patients with ankylosing spondylitis. This could be helpful in managing patients in clinical practice.

Taken together, these new developments signify that we are in an exciting era which will see improvements in our knowledge of the pathogenesis, course and prognosis of ankylosing spondylitis. For patients, the time has come when effective treatment is available to manage their disease.

Useful addresses

Assessment in Ankylosing
Spondylitis (ASAS) Working Group
mail@asas-group.org
www.asas-group.org

National Ankylosing Spondylitis
Society
PO Box 179
Mayfield
East Sussex
TN20 6ZL, UK
Tel: 01435 873527
Fax: 01435 873027
nass@nass.org.uk
www.nass.co.uk

Spondylitis Association of
America (SAA)
PO Box 5872
Sherman Oaks
CA 91413, USA
Tel: 800 777 8189
info@spondylitis.org

Index